# *Help Yourself*

# Help Yourself:
# The Beginner's Guide to Natural Medicine

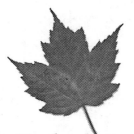

by Karolyn A. Gazella

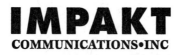
COMMUNICATIONS•INC

# Help Yourself:
# The Beginner's Guide to Natural Medicine

### by Karolyn A. Gazella

Copyright © 1995 IMPAKT Communications, Inc.
Library of Congress Catalog Card Number: 95-95161
ISBN 0-9647489-1-6

Cover Illustration by Lynn Poshepny
Cover Design by Karolyn A. Gazella

To order contact:

IMPAKT Communications, Inc.
P.O. Box 12496
Green Bay, WI  54307-2496
Credit card orders can call 1-800-477-2995
FAX (414) 499-3441
Quantity discounts available

# DEDICATION

This book is dedicated to the loving memory of my mom, Eunice Gazella, who passed away on January 6, 1995, at the age of 58. In her life she was a vibrant, giving person and in her death she remains an inspiration to all of us who loved her.

# CONTENTS

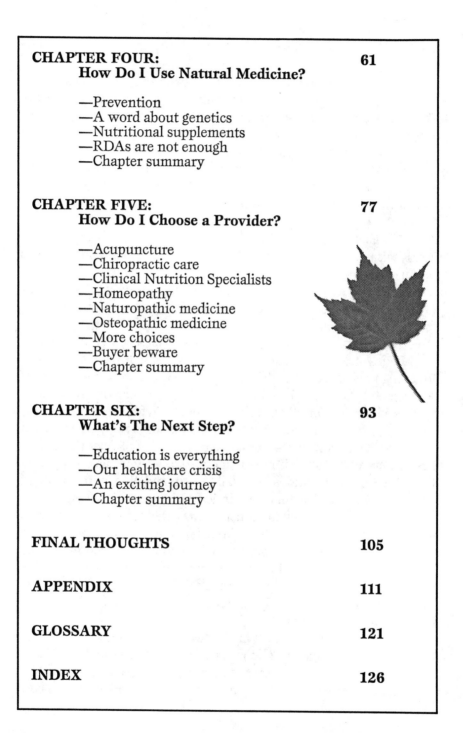

## ACKNOWLEDGMENTS

I am a very fortunate person. I have been supported by so many quality individuals, that to list them all here would not be feasible. But there are many who must be mentioned because their contribution to this book and my life has been immeasurable.

First, the many healthcare professionals that I have had the pleasure of working with over the years: Dr. Michael Murray, Dr. Judy Christianson, Dr. Herb Joyner Baye, Dr. Kevon Arthurs, Dr. Alan Gaby, Dr. Patrick Quillin, Dr. Jan McBarron, Dr. Steve Austin and his wife Cathy Hitchcock, Dr. Carolyn DeMarco, Dr. Alexander Schauss, Dr. Anthony Cichoke, and Dr. Charles Simone. Thanks to health writers Siri Khalsa and Ann Louise Gittleman C.N.S. for their contributions to our magazines.

My friends in the health food store business including: Sue Kranick of Bay Natural Foods in Green Bay, WI; Kathy Mazur and her store manager LuAnn Randolph from For The Good of It in Joliet, IL; and Vera Weido of Nature's Way in San Antonio, TX. Thanks for your support.

My dear friend and a talented writer, Frances FitzGerald, thanks for being there. Susan Reinfeldt, Kris Labutzke, and Sandy Mathy of American Medical Security for their friendship and support. To my good friend and mentor Terry Lemerond, president and founder of Enzymatic Therapy. To all of the great people of Enzymatic Therapy—I am proud to be associated with such a fine company. To all of the many fine businesses I have worked with over the years and who have supported IMPAKT Communications especially Kevin and Nancy Kohrman, of Kohrman Graphic Design, for their dedication and friendship.

A special thanks to Lynn Poshepny, the gifted artist and friend who did the illustration on the cover of this book.

To my family and the many friends who have helped me on my journey. To the people of IMPAKT Communications—Shelly Petska, our sales director, who helped so much with this book, your dedication and friendship is greatly appreciated; and Lisa Nischke, thanks for all of your hard work.

To Jackie Pederson, one of my biggest supporters and best friend, I love you dearly. Most of all, to my sister, Kathi Magee and her family Keith, Cody and Travis. Kathi has inspired me in so many ways. She is not only my sister, but also my business partner and one of my best friends. I appreciate your support and unconditional love.

Saving the best for last, I would like to thank all the readers of our three national magazines: *Health Counselor*, *Health Security*, and *The American Journal of Natural Medicine*. Your support is truly appreciated; after all, if it wasn't for you, there would be no IMPAKT Communications.

## FOREWARD
## by Michael T. Murray, N.D.

In *Help Yourself: The Beginner's Guide to Natural Medicine*, Karolyn Gazella has done a magnificent job of providing the guidance so that you can better understand the various natural healing techniques and how to find the practitioners who perform them. If you haven't consulted an alternative healthcare provider, this book will surely inspire you to do so.

More and more Americans are seeking "alternative" treatments. Although some view the increased popularity of alternative medicine as a sign of a medical revolution, I prefer to view it as an evolution. I believe what is currently viewed as alternative to many will soon become part of mainstream medicine. Karolyn Gazella is playing a major role in the integration of alternative medicine into the mainstream. In addition to this excellent guide, she is the editor and publisher of three very important national publications—*Health Counselor, Health Security*, and *The American Journal of Natural Medicine*—that are at the forefront of educating the public and healthcare professionals regarding the benefits of various "natural" medicines.

Why are so many people seeking alternative therapies? I think the obvious answer is that they are finding out that these natural treatments work! I also think that Americans are tired of being subservient to the will of their physician. They want to play a greater role in the direction of their healthcare. They want to explore options and educate themselves on what they can do besides take a pill that will likely do them more harm than good.

Modern medicine has not done a very good job at teaching people how to be healthy. The dominant medical model is really not a "healthcare" model, instead it is a "disease care" model that focuses on using drugs or surgery to promote health. This view is rapidly being replaced by a more rational model of health promotion where the focus is on what can be done to promote health rather than treat disease.

The focus of what is currently labeled as alternative medicine is health promotion, not disease treatment. Most alternative medical practitioners adhere to five time-tested medical principles. These principles serve as the foundation upon which the alternative healthcare provider practices, whether that practitioner is a naturopath, chiropractor, acupuncturist, nutritionist, or medical doctor.

**Principle 1: The healing power of nature.**

The body has considerable power to heal itself. It is the role of the physician or healer to facilitate and enhance this process, preferably, with the aid of natural, nontoxic therapies. Above all else, the physician or healer must do no harm.

**Principle 2: View the whole person.**

An individual must be viewed as a whole person composed of a complex interaction of physical, mental/emotional, spiritual, social, and other factors.

**Principle 3: Identify and treat the cause.**

It is important to seek the underlying cause of a disease rather than simply suppress the symptoms. Symptoms are viewed as expressions of the body's attempt to heal while the causes can spring from the physical, mental/emotional, and spiritual levels.

**Principle 4: The physician as teacher.**

A physician should be foremost a teacher. Educating, empowering, and motivating the patient to assume more personal responsibility for their health by adopting a healthy attitude, lifestyle, and diet.

**Principle 5: Prevention is the best cure.**

Prevention of disease is best accomplished through dietary and life habits which support health and prevent disease.

Undoubtedly, these natural principles of healing will persist throughout the future. By acting as a vital link in the evolution of medicine, these underlying principles of "good" medicine provide a bridge between the medicine of the past and the medicine of the future. Perhaps the famous words of Thomas Edison will turn out to be truly prophetic:

*"The doctor of the future will give no medicine, but will interest his patient in the care of the human frame, in diet and in the cause and prevention of disease."*

*Help Yourself: The Beginner's Guide to Natural Medicine* will help lead you to these physicians of the future today.

Michael T. Murray, N.D.
September 1995

# INTRODUCTION

## Good Health
## Begins With You!

I f you or someone you love has ever been faced with a serious illness, you found out first-hand just how important our health is to us. You will probably agree that our health is our most important asset. It's a gift that should be cherished and we should do everything in our power to protect it.

There was a time when I felt invincible. Although I have seen aunts and uncles and grandparents stricken with serious illness, I just never thought it could happen to me. Even when my only sister, who was 35-years-old at the time, was operated on for breast cancer in July 1994, I still thought it could never happen to me. Even when my mom passed away from terminal cancer just five months after my sister's operation, I still thought I was immune to serious illness. I was wrong! Less than three months after my mom's death, I found out I had ovarian cancer. Two days after my 33rd birthday, I had a complete hysterectomy due to the cancer. Today, I know I'm not invincible. However, I am happy to report that my prognosis is very good and I am feeling fantastic!

I have been studying and using natural medicines for more than six years. I have found that before and after my cancer, natural medicine has been an important part of my healthcare regimen. It's a choice that I'm glad I made. I have experienced both sides of the fence and have found tremendous benefit from each side. There needs to be both conventional as well as natural medicine in order for complete healing to take place. I have been thankful for the surgeon who removed my tumor and have really appreciated my natural medicine associates who have provided me with the proper natural treatment plan and the information I needed to get my body and mind back on track.

People have told me that I am very fortunate to be a health researcher and writer. I get to study illnesses and treatment options. Some of the very concepts I have studied over the years have helped my sister and me very much. One of the concepts that I have found to be extremely important is natural medicine.

Natural medicine has been catapulted to the forefront of our ailing healthcare system. According to a report featured in *The New England Journal of Medicine* (1994), one in three Americans is presently using some form of alternative healthcare, spending $14 billion a year. There is no question that what used to be a simmering interest among an isolated group of visionaries is now boiling over into mainstream America.

The American public is taking control. And if you are like most people, you are tired of ineffective, expensive medical treatments riddled with side effects and risk. You, like millions of others, are searching for alternatives in the area of disease prevention and treatment. What you will find during your search is a wealth of information regarding natural medicine. You, too, are likely to join the ranks of the countless Americans who educate themselves about all of their alternatives, including natural medicine.

So, what's all the fuss? What is natural medicine, anyway? And how do you even get started using the treatments, products and services provided by the natural medicine industry?

If you are interested in finding the answers to these and other important questions about natural medicine, you've come to the right place. *Help Yourself: The Beginner's Guide to Natural Medicine* will help you make sense of it all. The goal of this book is to help you take control of your health by teaching you how to incorporate natural medicine philosophies into your health program. It will lay the foundation for future good health and provide you with the basics of natural medicine. You will find the natural medicine treatment plans to be effective, less expensive, and safer than many of our conventional medical procedures. This book will also help clarify some of the key facts about natural medicine as well as destroy some of the myths about holistic healthcare providers and their services. You will get started on the road to empowerment, ready to take control of your health regardless of the present national healthcare climate.

Throughout the years, many people have written to me, telling me about how natural medicine has made a difference in their lives. I have had the privilege of working with and interviewing many extremely talented healthcare professionals, including the late Dr. Linus Pauling. I have personally experienced the power of many nutritional supplements. My sister and I are proud to be cancer survivors and we're excited to tell the world that natural medicine is an important part of our healing process.

Our healthcare system has much to offer us—and that includes natural medicine. If you are only familiar with conventional medical procedures and treatments, you are only getting part of the picture. This book is intended to provide you with introductory information about that missing link—natural medicine, holistic healthcare, alternative therapies. No matter what the label, the foundation is solid and the concepts and philosophies are strong.

Information is power. And you will learn that the power begins with you. By reading this book, you are making that important first step. Now, it's time you learned how you can save money while using effective, non-toxic alternative treatments. There is no question that natural medicine offers you a viable alternative.

It is important to emphasize that the purpose of this book is educational. The information provided is not intended as advice for self-diagnosis or self-treatment. I recommend you consult a qualified healthcare professional before adopting any dramatic changes in dietary guidelines or nutritional or medical treatments. For this reason, I have included advice on how to pick a qualified healthcare professional.

Congratulations for taking such a strong interest in your health. Soon, you will no longer be a beginner, and you will be ready for the next step. You can expect an exciting and interesting journey!

# CHAPTER ONE

## What is Natural Medicine?

I t's been called many things: Alternative. Holistic. Complementary. Comprehensive. And, yes, even quackery. Even the term "natural medicine" is too limiting, because it's so much more than just "medicine." It's a philosophy that involves many variables.

Natural medicine views health as a puzzle. When even one piece is missing, the puzzle is incomplete. Regardless of what you may have heard about natural medicine, there are no magic bullets. We all know that it takes more than one piece to complete the puzzle. We also know that our health can be considered one of the most complicated puzzles of all. So, it only makes sense that there are many pieces needed. The completed puzzle is, of course, optimum health.

One of the most important concepts about natural medicine and holistic healthcare is that you are in control. With help, you can decide which piece of the puzzle is missing and how you want to fill in the gap. It all begins and ends with you. After all, it's your body. And the power to heal lies within you.

### From concept to care

Natural medicine is an umbrella term representing a plethora of services, products, and treatments. Everything from dietary changes to detoxification procedures can be called holistic or fall into the category of natural medicine. Here are some tidbits of information about just some of the opportunities available under the umbrella:

- Chiropractic care—In 1980, there were one million patients utilizing chiropractic medicine. Today there are 19 million.
- Nutritional supplements (i.e. vitamins, herbal extracts, etc.)—In 1994 alone, Americans spent well over $700 million on herbal medicines obtained from health food stores. Add to that the interest in all nutritional supplements and you have a nearly four and one-half billion dollar industry.
- Acupuncture—Three thousand United States physicians use acupuncture in their practice, up from 500 ten years ago. Nine to 12 million acupuncture treatments are performed in the United States each year according to the Food and Drug Administration.
- Homeopathy—Practiced widely in Europe, this respected form of medicine has been recognized in the United States for nearly 200 years.
- Ayurvedic medicine—This ancient form of medicine originated in India and is gaining popularity in the United States.

(These are just a few of the treatments, products, and services provided by natural medicine. For a more complete list with definitions, refer to page 16.)

All of these treatment modalities, and the others associated with natural medicine, have one thing in common—their philosophy. Natural medicine providers and users believe that the power to heal lies within the human body. If you provide your body with the proper tools, it can and will heal itself, naturally, without synthetic drugs or invasive surgery. The natural medicine concept believes that drugs and surgery should only be used when the body is in crisis and cannot defend itself properly. There is a strong emphasis on proactive health-care and disease prevention. Natural medicine looks less at symptoms and more at etiology—what is causing the symptoms in the first place. By treating the actual cause, natural medicine provides a long-term solution to short-term symptoms.

Henry David Thoreau wrote: *"Nature is doing her best each moment to make us well. She exists for no other end. Do not resist. With the least inclination to be well, we should not be sick."*

The power of nature is another common theme among holistic healthcare providers and their treatments. Herbal medicines, for example, stimulate different body functions to help you stay well or become well again. According to Michael T. Murray, N.D., noted author and natural medicine researcher, the new natural medicine view is surfacing as the rational alternative. Dr. Murray believes the era of self-empowerment is beginning and natural medicine is a key component of that era. Here are characteristics of the new healthcare paradigm as taken from Dr. Murray's latest book, *Natural Alternatives to Over-the-Counter and Prescription Drugs*:

- Natural medicine is concerned with the whole person.
- The body and the mind are interconnected.
- The emphasis is on achieving health rather than simply treating symptoms.
- There is an integrated approach to treatment rather than specialization.
- There is a focus on diet, lifestyle, and preventive measures.
- The physician's attitude of caring and empathy are critical to the healing process.
- The physician is a partner in the process.
- The patient is in charge of his/her own healthcare choices.
- There is more focus on how the patient is feeling.

The change is already taking place. In fact, many medical organizations that have in the past spoken out against natural medicine are now endorsing the concepts. Most physicians today recommend that we eat more fiber and reduce sugar and fat intake—advice natural medicine practitioners have been giving for decades. Many conventional physicians now advocate regular exercise and even vitamin supplements.

"In most instances, the natural alternative offers significant benefit over standard medical practices," concluded Dr. Murray.

In light of this renewed interest, organizations (see the appendix of this book for a list) have been established to get the word out to physicians and their patients about the benefits of natural medicine. There seems to be a new understanding of "alternative" medicine and an immediate need for accurate information.

"In the face of an increasingly inadequate system of conventional medicine, a growing number of people are turning to alternative medicine to address their needs," according to the popular reference book, *Alternative Medicine: The definitive guide*. "The general public is starting to recognize the effectiveness of alternative medicine's

approach to health, which blends body and mind, science and experience, and traditional and cross cultural avenues of diagnosis and treatment."

Because the holistic view concentrates so fully on body function,
it's important to have a basic understanding of how our bodies work.

### A quick lesson in body function

When discussing the important components of natural medicine,
body function is at the top of the list. Natural medicine proponents
believe the human body has phenomenal power to heal itself. Your body
is continuously communicating with you through various signals.
Learning to recognize those signals is the first step in preventing and
treating illness. But first, we need to review the key components of the
body.

Let's start with the **immune system**. It's a great place to start
because a healthy immune system is absolutely critical in maintaining
good health. You can never overestimate the importance of immune
system function. Examples of some signals that a weak immune
system will send to you are:

- frequent bouts of the flu and colds
- low energy levels
- allergies to food, dust, chemicals, etc.
- difficulty dealing with stress
- infections

Your immune system is your only defense against many illnesses.
Your immune system is equipped with all of the necessary weapons
to keep you healthy. T-cells are white blood cells that are the key fighters
on the immune system's defense team. T-cells mature in the thymus,
which has frequently been called the master gland of immunity. That's
why it's so important to keep your thymus gland healthy, so it can keep
you healthy. The thymus is critical in helping T-cells become mature
and effective. The thymus gland is located in the middle of your chest
above your heart. (We will discuss thymus extract and its effect on the
immune system in more detail in a later chapter.)

Lymph nodes are meeting rooms for immune cells. That's where
T-cells and other important immune soldiers congregate until they are
needed. When they are called upon, they travel in lymph, which is a
clear fluid that circulates throughout the body.

The spleen, like the lymph nodes, is also an important gathering place for immune cells. While in the spleen, immune cells work to rid the body of antigens, which are the enemy. Antigens identify "bad" cells from "good" cells and then they stimulate the immune response, which destroys bad cells. When immune cells target antigens, they kick their army into action, offering you protection from a wide variety of conditions.

Immune system cells enter the bloodstream and patrol the body. They work to kill foreign antigens and then gradually make their way back to the lymph nodes or the spleen. The immune system patrol occurs constantly and is your body's way of getting rid of foreign, dangerous materials.

Immune cells actually communicate with each other searching out and destroying foreign invaders as quickly and efficiently as possible. T-cells and B-cells are the most important lymphocytes in the body. They work to regulate immune response and help attack and kill bad cells. It is this process that helps protect us from immune system illnesses, including very serious conditions such as AIDS, cancer and hepatitis.

The immune system is a fascinating component of the human body. Volumes could be written on this subject alone; however, the most important aspect to remember is that if we keep our body's immune system healthy, it will keep us healthy. Unfortunately, many aspects of our Western lifestyle can hinder this process. Environmental toxins, pesticides, tobacco smoke, highly processed foods, and stress are just a few examples of immune compromisers. For this reason, we should take extra care when trying to keep our immune system healthy (we'll discuss this more in later chapters).

Along with the immune system, you should know about your **central nervous system**. Of course, the commander of our central nervous system is our brain. The immune system and the central nervous system are linked in many ways. One of the main links is with the adrenal glands. As the brain responds to stress, hormones from the adrenal glands are released. Although these hormones feel they are helping the body deal with the stress, they actually reduce lymphocyte (immune cell) activity.

Research indicates that the brain communicates with the immune system by sending messages that can either enhance or endanger our health. There is no debating the strong connection between how we think and how we feel. The subliminal dance between our brain and our immune system may, in fact, determine how many healthy steps we will take. We'll talk more about this important connection later.

Your central nervous system controls your brain function and nerve signals. Just like your immune system, your central nervous system will send you many warning signals when things just aren't quite right, including, but surely not limited to:

- depression
- anxiety
- lethargy
- dizziness
- poor memory

It is clear that the central nervous system, like the immune system, can be negatively affected by environmental toxins, which can cause many of the symptoms listed above. We live in a very toxic world. Since World War II, there have been about 70,000 new chemicals introduced to the United States. Each year, the United States produces an estimated nine billion pounds of formaldehyde, which has been shown to cause cancer in animals. According to the California Public Interest Research Group, the United States produces 250 billion pounds of synthetic chemicals every year.

Everything from lead in our drinking water to radon in the basement can cause problems for susceptible people. Pesticides, asbestos, and cigarette smoke are also very dangerous contaminants that can lead to serious health problems. There are about 4,000 chemicals in tobacco smoke, 43 of which are known carcinogens (cancer-causing agents). The Environmental Protection Agency has estimated that about 20,000 cancer deaths occur each year due to radon gas seepage in the home and about 6,000 cancer deaths are caused each year by other indoor air pollutants.

Never underestimate the damage environmental pollutants can have on your health. Typically, the key organ most commonly affected by such environmental toxins is the brain—the focal point for our central nervous system.

Fortunately, your body has a method of eliminating toxins. The **detoxification system** is your body's way of getting rid of anything that's harmful. Detoxification is a continual process for the human

# Detoxification

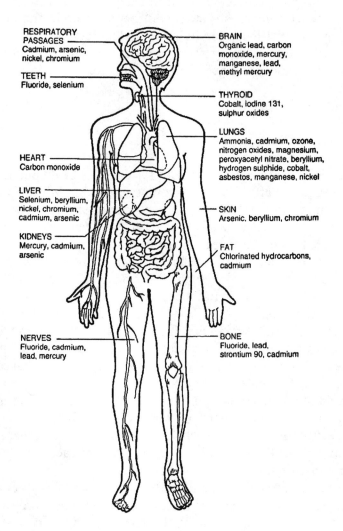

RESPIRATORY
PASSAGES
Cadmium, arsenic,
nickel, chromium

TEETH
Fluoride, selenium

HEART
Carbon monoxide

LIVER
Selenium, beryllium,
nickel, chromium,
cadmium, arsenic

KIDNEYS
Mercury, cadmium,
arsenic

NERVES
Fluoride, cadmium,
lead, mercury

BRAIN
Organic lead, carbon
monoxide, mercury,
manganese, lead,
methyl mercury

THYROID
Cobalt, iodine 131,
sulphur oxides

LUNGS
Ammonia, cadmium, ozone,
nitrogen oxides, magnesium,
peroxyacetyl nitrate, beryllium,
hydrogen sulphide, cobalt,
asbestos, manganese, nickel

SKIN
Arsenic, beryllium, chromium

FAT
Chlorinated hydrocarbons,
cadmium

BONE
Fluoride, lead,
strontium 90, cadmium

Main targets of major air pollutants.

—Source: *Encyclopedia of Natural Medicine*
by Michael Murray, N.D. and Joseph Pizzorno, N.D.

body. The efficiency of this process depends largely on your overall health. The healthier you are, the more effectively you will be able to rid your body of harmful toxins. The reverse is also true. If you are not in good health, your body will be even more sensitive to everyday toxins. This is important because, as mentioned previously, many toxins have been shown to erode our health. Environmental illnesses and other conditions associated with these toxins, such as chronic fatigue syndrome, attention deficit disorder, and many others are plaguing America.

In addition to the detoxification process, our **digestive system** is still another key contributor to our overall health. There is no question that proper digestion is absolutely necessary for good health. Poor digestion can actually cause many serious illnesses. The problem with poor digestion is really twofold:

1. When our food is poorly digested, we are not getting all of the benefits from the food causing deficiencies, and
2. Incompletely digested food molecules can be absorbed into our bloodstream and cause food allergies, depression and various other problems.

Symptoms of poor digestion can include:
- abdominal pain
- altered bowel function
- frequent bouts of gas, indigestion and heartburn
- nausea, diarrhea, or anorexia

Keeping your digestive system working efficiently will help keep your body on track.

From digestion, we move up to respiration. Our lungs are the key organ within our **respiratory system**. At one point or another, we have all had a cold that settles in our chest, making it difficult to breathe. Although the common cold is not deadly, long-term unhealthy lung function is. The lungs are responsible for exchanging carbon dioxide for oxygenated blood. Oxygen deficiency can cause many serious problems.

Serious illnesses affecting the respiratory system include, but are not limited to, asthma, bronchitis, pneumonia, and lung cancer. Keeping our lungs healthy and working properly is an important part of our healthcare plan. Of course, one of the key ways you can do this is by avoiding cigarette smoke.

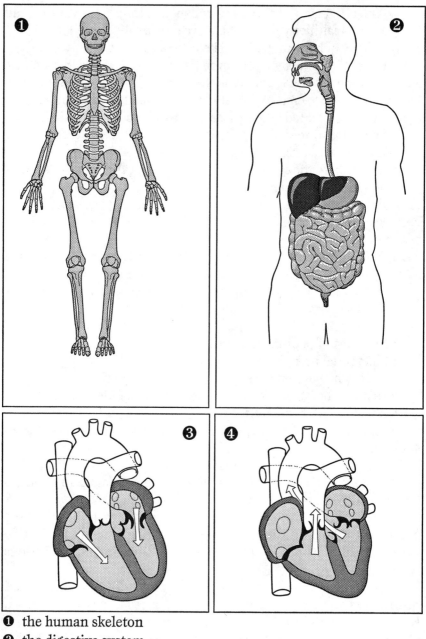

❶ the human skeleton
❷ the digestive system
❸ & ❹ action of the heart pumping blood

Here are the other key areas of the body that we need to keep functioning properly in order to obtain optimum health:
- Muscles and bones
- The sensory organs (sight, taste, smell, hearing, touch)
- Reproductive organs
- The endocrine glands (adrenals, pancreas, ovaries in women, testes in men, pituitary, thyroid, and hypothalamus in the brain)

At the "heart" of all of these important body functions is our **cardiovascular system**. It is clear that an unhealthy cardiovascular system is not only dangerous, it's deadly. Heart disease is the number one killer of Americans today. It is clear that keeping our cardiovascular system in good shape is critical. An estimated 65 million Americans have some form of heart disease. And it is important to remember that although heart disease typically rears its head later in life (age 50 or older), it actually takes years to develop. What you do when you are 20 years old will determine how well you live when you're 50 or 60 years old. And if you are over 50 years old, you must make necessary lifestyle changes right away.

Here are the major risk factors for developing heart disease:
- smoking
- high blood pressure
- high cholesterol
- obesity (more than 20 pounds over your normal weight—refer to the weight chart in Chapter Three)
- family history of heart disease
- sedentary lifestyle (very little exercise)
- high stress

Recognizing the risk factors and developing a plan to reduce or eliminate those factors will help you avoid heart disease.

To say the human body is a very complex unit is quite an understatement. Although you don't need to hold a medical degree, a basic understanding of how our bodies work is important in understanding the big picture. When it comes to health, we need to see the completed puzzle before we can keep the pieces together. Recognizing that we have the power to keep the puzzle together or put the pieces back together if necessary is the first step in understanding natural medicine. After you realize you have the power, it's necessary to learn about the products, treatments and services that are available to you.

## Products and services

Just as with any healthcare system, there are specific natural medicine tools used to promote better health. Conventional medicine uses surgery, over-the-counter and prescription medicines, and many expensive, high-tech tests and techniques. Natural medicine practitioners use the following treatments, products, and services to heal their patients:

- Acupuncture—The use of thin, disposable needles to stimulate specific points in the body to renew energetic balance.
- Ayurvedic medicine—An ancient form of treatment involving diet, detoxification, exercise, herbal medicine, and meditation used to treat a wide variety of chronic conditions including arthritis, asthma, allergies, etc.
- Biofeedback—Training of the involuntary nervous system using sound devices to treat conditions such as stress, migraines, asthma, and high blood pressure.
- Body work (massage, reiki, rolfing, etc.)—Physical manipulation to provide balance in the body, reduce stress in the muscles, and help alleviate many illnesses associated with body structure.
- Chelation therapy—Use of an intravenous solution to remove heavy metals and toxins from the body and most commonly used to treat heart conditions.
- Chiropractic care—By using spinal manipulation and dietary and lifestyle counselling virtually any chronic condition can be treated with chiropractic care.
- Comprehensive patient questionnaire—A thorough evaluation of health history and present symptoms and concerns.
- Detoxification therapy—Various forms of detoxification, including fasting, hydrotherapy, and juicing help rid the body of chemicals and pollutants to help facilitate a return to good health.
- Diagnostic tests—Blood tests, urinalysis, hair analysis etc.
- Guided imagery—Capitalizing on the power of the mind, mental pictures are created to help stimulate a positive physical response.
- Glandular therapy—Like heals like. By giving a product that contains gland extracts of the same organ you are having difficulty with will help the body heal itself (i.e. liver, spleen, thymus, etc.).
- Herbal medicines—Plant substances which have been shown to

have medicinal effects are used to treat a wide variety of health conditions including arthritis, immune system disorders, heart disease, and other chronic illnesses.

- Homeopathy—Miniscule traces of a medicinal substance(s) that would cause the same symptoms of the condition in a healthy person is used to stimulate the body's healing processes.
- Hydrotherapy—The use of various hot and cold water treatments for a wide range of digestive, circulatory, and respiratory conditions.
- Hypnotherapy—A method used to tap into a person's unconscious mind to help facilitate the treatment of a variety of conditions including depression, anxiety, eating disorders, etc.
- Nutritional and psychological counseling—Working with the patient by providing nutritional advice and psychological support.
- Nutritional supplements—Vitamins, minerals, amino acids, glandulars, herbs, and other nutrients either alone or in combination with each other to make up a formulation to support body function or treat a wide variety of illnesses including female problems, immune system disorders, blood pressure, etc.

As you can see, there are many holistic healthcare services, treatments, and products available through natural medicine practitioners or as self-care items you purchase over-the-counter. Don't let the list of these "unknown" treatments intimidate you. Don't expect to learn them all at once. Pick one or two that you find the most interesting to study first.

The appendix lists valuable sources of information about natural medicine practitioners and services. You will find the information these organizations provide quite helpful. Your local health food store is also an excellent source of information. Many health food stores have an extensive selection of books and literature. Many stores carry our *Health Counselor* magazine and give it to their customers as a gift to help keep them informed on the latest advances in natural medicine.

## History repeats

The use of natural medicine to help the body heal itself is certainly not a new concept. Natural medicine and the treatments, services, and products described earlier have a very long-standing tradition and a solid track record, with some dating back to the beginning of time.

Naturopathic medicine, for example, has been recognized by the American medical profession since 1902. Homeopathic medicine has an extensive history here in the United States and Europe. In fact, by the close of the 19th century, there were 22 homeopathic medical schools, more than 100 homeopathic hospitals, and about 15 percent of the physician population was practicing homeopathy. Unfortunately, in 1910 the government began using American Medical Association (AMA) guidelines for the funding of medical schools. Because the newly established guidelines favored the AMA standards, competing medical schools, such as those devoted to homeopathy, were financially crippled. Today, however, we are finding that history has not been forgotten.

Before there were antibiotics, there was natural medicine. Before there was aspirin, there was natural medicine. And long before there was open heart surgery or balloon angioplasty, there was natural medicine.

There are still some people who dismiss natural medicine and think of it as bizarre or useless. I wonder if those same people realize that more than 25 percent of the prescription drugs in this country are made from herbs? Do they realize that homeopathy, for example, has been used successfully for nearly 200 years?

The scientific effectiveness of herbal medicines is so strong that Dr. Michael Murray states, "If current standardization techniques had been available earlier in this century, it is possible that the majority of our current prescription drugs would be crude herbal extracts instead of isolated and modified active constituents." The herbal standardization process is discussed in much more detail in a later chapter.

Natural medicine is a staple in many European healthcare communities. It is a first line of treatment and readily available in pharmacies and doctor's offices throughout Europe. Many countries, such as India, China and Greece, rely heavily on natural medicine.

The medicine of the past is now becoming the medicine of the future. Standing firm on a foundation of historic use, scientific evidence, and a future filled with new technology and renewed interest, natural medicine is no longer an alternative. It is a mainstay for many individuals.

**The philosophy**

Knowledge about body function is very important to natural medicine. People who believe in natural medicine believe in the power of the human body. The body has the ability to stay healthy and regain good health. Give your body what it needs and it won't let you down. Abuse your body and chances are, you will suffer the consequences.

One of the primary aspects of the natural medicine philosophy that many people find so appealing is that the least toxic treatments are employed first. The natural medicine community takes the Hippocratic oath—"first, do no harm"—very seriously.

Giving you and your body some credit and control, is the other key philosophy behind natural medicine. People who believe in natural medicine believe they have the power and understand that true healing lies within. Knowing how to stimulate this power is the most important aspect of natural healing. This is the most potent medicine of all—it's a healing you will discover as you study natural medicine.

Truly holistic healthcare programs believe in a comprehensive approach. This approach combines conventional and natural medicines and recognizes the power of the human body and the mind that controls it. There is no doubt that there is not only room for both, but that both are necessary for optimum health.

Using all of the healthcare options available to you, beginning with the least toxic, is what natural medicine is all about. It is a concept that more and more people are adopting. It is a philosophy that is no longer "alternative," but mainstream.

**Chapter summary**

We've learned that no matter what you label it, natural medicine has a respected history of use and has become a viable first choice in the treatment of many illnesses. It is also a staple of any comprehensive health prevention program.

What is natural medicine?

- It is a philosophy that puts you, the patient, in charge of your health.
- It is a complex group of products, services, treatments and concepts.
- It recognizes the power within and works to capitalize on that energy.

• It has a long history of use and is backed by scientific evidence.

Learning to listen to your body and giving it what it needs is an important part of natural medicine. We'll explore this concept more in chapters to follow. Until then, let's take a closer look at safety and science.

# CHAPTER TWO

# Is Natural Medicine Safe?

Our health is the cornerstone of our life. Without our health, our dreams, goals, and possible future accomplishments merely become emotional torture as we are unable to attain them. If we picture what our life would be like without vibrant health or the health of our close friends and family, we see a very bleak picture. That's why the safety of the products and services we use to gain better health or maintain optimum health is so important. We don't want anything to jeopardize our health or our recovery.

As we learned earlier, "First, do no harm," is the anchor of the natural medicine philosophy. But, really, how safe are natural products, services, or treatments? Who says they're safe? And what about the science of natural medicine—is there a strong scientific foundation that natural medicine stands upon? Or is the logic flawed and distorted?

We'll answer those questions and more, but first let's take a look at why natural medicine has become so popular.

## The old becomes new again

As discussed in Chapter One, natural medicine has a long history of use. Today, it is clear that what was once "old" has now become new again. It's been called a paradigm shift in healthcare because of our new view of an old model. But whatever you call it, there is no question that there is renewed interest in the treatment practices of "yesterday."

You will often hear natural medicine practitioners and patients talk about "historical use." This refers to how the treatment or product (herb or nutrient, for example) has been used in the past, which can oftentimes be traced back thousands of years. This term also refers to how these natural treatments have been used historically in a variety of cultures for specific conditions and illnesses. Many natural medicine practitioners have studied historical use extensively.

Although historical use does not equal scientific validation, it does provide us with some important insight into safety and effectiveness of many natural medicines. It also provides a key advantage over conventional drugs and procedures. Many conventional drugs and procedures do not have any "historical" use. In fact, many drugs on the market today have absolutely no guarantees regarding long-term usage. If you look in the *Physicians Desk Reference* (PDR), which is the medical doctor's pharmaceutical bible, you will notice that many common prescription drugs clearly indicate that there have not been tests or studies done on the ramifications of long-term usage. Often, the side effects associated with extended use of many prescription drugs are at best unknown, and at worst, deadly.

Ritalin®, for example, is a commonly prescribed medication for children with attention deficit hyperactivity disorder. According to information I have been provided by readers, friends and other health publications, this drug is clearly overprescribed. And, unfortunately, parents are often not getting the full picture. For example, according to the PDR, Ritalin "should not be used in children under six years, since safety and efficacy (effectiveness) in this age group have not been established." I personally know of quite a few children under age six who have either been on Ritalin or got started on Ritalin before age six. Even more startling, is that the safety of long-term usage of Ritalin is really unknown. Again, according to the PDR, "Sufficient data on safety and efficacy of long-term use of Ritalin in children are not yet available." The PDR warns that Ritalin usage can result in the development of Tourette's Syndrome and can stunt the growth of children. And yet, Ritalin usage is increasing dramatically. During a national newscast regarding a shortage of Ritalin in 1994, it was reported that sales have increased by more than 33 percent in that year alone.

The overprescribing of Ritalin is a problem in our present society. Let's take my nephew, for example. I may be prejudiced, but I think my nephews are extremely bright, creative young people. Teachers of one of my nephews told my sister that his energy and enthusiasm (qualities that I just love about him), "could be a sign of attention deficit hyperactivity disorder." Their recommendation: You guessed it— Ritalin. My sister, of course, set them straight. Instead of putting him on Ritalin, which would have been the "easiest" option, she chose to work with him and channel his energy. His report cards have been great and he is a joy to be around—instead of a zombie, like so many other children who are given Ritalin. There is no question that Ritalin serves an important purpose and it means the difference between learning and not learning for some children; however, it should not be our **first** option, but rather our **last** resort.

Another pharmaceutical example of unknown long-term usage of an approved drug is Prozac®, a popular anti-depressant. While Prozac, as well as Ritalin, can be vital to some individuals, the overprescribing of this drug by some healthcare providers has been under attack by the media. Although Prozac is clearly an antidepressant, it has been prescribed for conditions other than depression including weight loss and premenstrual syndrome (PMS). "Prozac is now being used to treat mild to moderate PMS in spite of troublesome side effects, including insomnia, nausea, and fatigue," according to Dr. Carolyn DeMarco. "The limited evidence to date shows only half of the women with very severe PMS respond moderately well to Prozac. Nondrug methods should always be fully explored first."

Unfortunately, like Ritalin, Prozac is sometimes employed as the first and only choice. Regarding long-term usage of Prozac, the PDR warns, "There is no body of evidence available to answer the question of how long the patient treated with Prozac should remain on it." Sounds like unsure science to me.

In contrast, the historical use of natural medicine products and treatments provides us with a pretty clear picture of safety. When a product or service has been used for decades, sometimes centuries, we can draw some pretty positive conclusions about safety. In fact, safety is one key reason why many individuals turn to natural medicine in the first place.

When asked why an individual chose natural medicine, the response is usually one or more of these:

• I wasn't getting any better.

- I was concerned about the long-term side effects of the drug(s) my doctor was recommending.
- I didn't feel my doctor listened enough or really cared about me.
- I felt my doctor was merely treating the symptoms without taking the time to get to the heart of my problem.
- I wanted to take more control of my own health.
- I was sick and tired of feeling sick and tired all of the time.
- I wanted to concentrate on prevention and ways to stay healthy.

So, the natural medicine advocate has learned how to educate themselves, just as you are doing by reading this book. And they discover that safety is one of the most important advantages of natural medicine.

### Harmful healthcare

There is no question that many drugs and conventional procedures have saved countless lives. The positive effects some drugs have on human health should not be ignored. After all, surgery to remove my tumor probably saved my life.

However, that's only half of the story. The damaging effects drugs and some conventional medical practices can have on an individual's body function and nutritional status should not be overlooked.

Let's take a look at a few examples of how conventional medical therapy can possibly do more harm than good:

1. **Overuse of antibiotics.** It has been shown conclusively that overuse of antibiotics not only kills off the bad bacteria but the good bacteria as well, causing people to become susceptible to chronic yeast infections. Overuse of antibiotics can also create a destructive immu-

---

After a seven-year study, the Congressional Office of Technology Assessment said in a report that among 241 American-made drugs sold in developing countries, 68 percent had labels with medically important omissions or additions. In the worst cases, potentially fatal side effects were left off the label, or new, unsupported claims to the drugs were added.

—*New York Times*, May 21, 1993

nity, whereby new "mutant" cells are created that will not respond to the antibiotic. In addition, antibiotics cause deficiencies of vitamin B12, folic acid, vitamin K, vitamin B2, and vitamin B1, according to natural medicine researcher Cass Igram, M.D.

2. **Surgery for localized prostate cancer.** According to the *Journal of the American Medical Association* (JAMA, May 26, 1993), radical prostatectomy (prostate removal) and radiation therapy for localized prostate cancer may not be the best treatment choice. JAMA researchers found that "watchful waiting" (i.e. no treatment at all) provides the patient with the same chance of survival with an improved quality of life compared to the surgery. Common complications of surgery and radiation include impotence and incontinence. Even though surgery and radiation have been used to treat localized prostate cancer for decades, the JAMA article revealed that only one randomized clinical trial had been done to evaluate the effectiveness of these treatments. The researchers concluded that if the same standards of safety and effectiveness for drug approval was used for surgery and radiation, neither of these treatments would be approved for localized prostate surgery.

3. **Chemotherapy and breast cancer.** *The New England Journal of Medicine* recently reported that when continuous chemotherapy was compared to no treatment at all in 250 women with breast cancer, the results showed that the chemotherapy did not improve survival rates. In fact, the chemotherapy was shown to have significantly decreased the quality of the life of those patients getting the treatment. Chemotherapy has been shown to cause damage to the immune system, kidney function, and liver resulting in many serious side effects. In general, chemotherapy is a very serious, dangerous drug. In fact, a poll of oncologists (cancer doctors who prescribe chemotherapy) revealed that if they got cancer, they would refuse the chemotherapy treatments.

4. **Heart medications.** Some heart medications have been clearly shown to actually do more harm than good. In a report published in the *New England Journal of Medicine* (November 21, 1991) when "compared to a placebo (fake pill), milrinone therapy resulted in a 28 percent increase in mortality from all causes and a 34 percent increase in cardiovascular mortality." Clofibrate, another heart medication, was proven to result in a 44 percent higher mortality rate when compared

## Pharmaceutical Facts

These facts taken from the Citizens For Health Newsletter (Winter 1992-93) show how the prices of prescription drugs have become almost unbearable:

- The inflation rate for all drugs sold in the United States rose 152 percent from 1980 to 1990.

- The cost of the most commonly used drugs by the elderly jumped eight times over the past six years.

- The cost of Naprosyn, a common arthritis medication, rose ten times in seven years.

- The cost of Inderal, a heart medication, rose 129 percent is six years.

- The top 15 drugs sold in the United States went up 192 percent in only three years.

- Because Medicare does not pay for prescription drugs, in 1987 alone, 64 percent of drug costs were out-of-pocket expenses.

- Synthroid, a thyroid replacement drug, rose 110 percent from 1985 to 1991, even though its formulation did not change at all during that time.

- Currently the United States leads the world in the cost of prescription drugs; drug costs are 32 percent higher in the United States than Canada; a United States consumer spending $400 on pharmaceuticals would spend $159 in Belgium and even less in Mexico for the same drugs.

- In 1991, the top twenty drug manufacturer's profit margins were nearly five times greater than that of the Fortune 500 companies.

to a placebo. And finally, Plendil, a channel blocking drug, had a laundry list of side effects listed in its ad in the *New England Journal of Medicine* promoting its use for heart disease. In addition to the numerous side effects at a dose of only five milligrams, the small print read: Plendil's "safety in patients with heart failure has not been established." There is no question that in these cases especially, the healthier choice would have been to avoid drug treatment altogether.

These are just a few of the many examples of the unsafe medical treatments and drugs that are being employed by our conventional healthcare system. We are often told that just because something is labeled "natural," doesn't mean it's safe. I would like to also propose that just because something is presently being used in our conventional medical system, also does not make it safe.

This seems to illustrate one of the key reasons more people are incorporating natural medicine into their health regimen. According to health writer Frances FitzGerald, there is a growing dissatisfaction with orthodox medicine among the American people. "Although the medical establishment has made enormous strides, sometimes the cure appears to be more harmful than the condition itself," reported Frances in *Health Counselor* magazine.

An article featured in a 1991 issue of the *New England Journal of Medicine* reported that in 1984, 98,609 patients were harmed and 13,451 patients were killed by standard hospital therapy in New York State alone. More recent reports indicate those numbers are on the rise. In 1990, the Centers for Disease Control and Prevention reported that there were 5,000 deaths directly caused by prescription drugs in that year. During the last decade, published estimates in medical journals reported that more than 500,000 Americans died from reactions to FDA-approved drugs, while they were in hospitals under medical supervision.

And then there's NutraSweet™, a brand-name sweetener presently used in well over 2,500 food items. In 1990 alone, nearly 80 percent of the 6,500 complaints received by the FDA from consumers were directed toward this artificial sweetener. NutraSweet (generically known as aspartame) has been shown to cause a number of serious health conditions including epileptic seizures.

In addition, a report by the United States Office of Technology Assessment submitted to Congress found that nearly 80 percent of all conventional medical therapies lack sufficient proof of effectiveness, including hundreds of devices approved by the FDA, and many common surgical procedures including angioplasty (for the heart) and carotid endarterectomies (removing obstructions from the artery).

All of these examples of problems with our conventional medical system help to illustrate that no form of medicine is without problems or concerns. Furthermore, it's understandable why more and more individuals are going the natural route before undertaking serious long-term prescription drug use or subjecting themselves to certain medical procedures.

### Safety first

For those in the conventional medical fields who so adamantly oppose natural medicine—usually because of safety—I contend that those who live in glass houses should not throw stones. In other words, unless their medications and treatments are completely without risk, they should have an open mind about other alternatives.

Abram Hoffer, M.D., Ph.D. is one of the leading researchers in the area of natural medicine. His scientific and clinical work is extensive and impressive. Here is what Dr. Hoffer has to say about the safety of natural substances: "...vitamins which are safe even in large doses have not been acceptable to the medical profession, and their negative side effects have been consistently exaggerated and over-emphasized, to the point that many of these so-called toxicities have been invented, without there being any scientific evidence that these side effects are real." Dr. Hoffer contends that we should take negative publicity about natural medicine with a grain of salt, for it just may be fiction rather than fact.

Whenever discussing natural medicine, opponents of the treatments often cite safety as a key concern. The fact is, however, natural medicine is quite safe. Obviously, no medical treatment is without some risk; however, the risks of natural medical treatments, products, and services are typically far less than many comparative conventional medical treatments, products, and services. The bottom line is that the natural alternatives have been proven to be much safer than their conventional counterpart in most cases.

In 1993, Citizens for Health, a nonprofit citizen advocacy group, reviewed a decade's worth of annual reports released by the 72 reporting centers of the American Association of Poison Control Centers, studies published in the *Journal of Emergency Medicine*, and the AMA's physician reporting system instituted in 1986. They found no reports of any deaths due to vitamin usage. "This suggests that dietary supplements have an extraordinary record of safety, particularly when you consider that well over 100 million Americans of all ages and health conditions consume these products each year," concluded Alexander Schauss, Ph.D., of Citizens for Health.

"It is ironic that an agency of government (the FDA) so concerned with public safety approves transplanting a baboon heart into a heart patient, while vigorously lobbying (with taxpayer money) to regulate coenzyme Q-10 (CoQ10), a substance found naturally in cells that could prevent many from needing such a surgery," explained Dr. Schauss. *(As a side note about CoQ10, I have found it to make a world of difference in my health and energy levels. CoQ10 is not a stimulant, but it is vital to the health of our cells, including our immune cells. I take a 100 mg tablet—Twin Labs brand—every morning.)*

In 1990, the CDC confirmed the safety of nutritional supplements. They reported only one death caused by vitamins in ten years. That particular death has since been refuted by nutritional experts.

"The limited data available suggests that adverse reactions to drugs are far more common than adverse reactions to pharmacological (large) dosages of nutrients," explained physician, researcher, author, and professor, Melvyn Werbach, M.D. According to Dr. Werbach, drugs are more toxic because they are foreign substances in the body. In contrast, "the absorption and metabolism of nutrients proceed according to physiological mechanisms that have developed and are continuous action for that very purpose," explained Dr. Werbach.

Unfortunately, the issue of safety is oftentimes not the issue at all. The politics of medicine have made it extremely difficult for natural medicine to proceed forward. It requires more than 250 million dollars to conduct the extensive clinical, double-blind studies required for FDA drug approval. The FDA also requires the study of a specific component, rather than a group of components, which is nearly impossible for herbs, for example, because they are made up of many synergistic parts that make up the whole. In addition, herbs and nutrients are natural substances and cannot be patented. So, if a company did spend the millions of dollars on getting approval, they could not patent the product, so any other manufacturer could market the same product in the same way. That's why pharmaceutical companies try to determine the exact active component of a plant. They then isolate that component, synthetically manufacture it as a drug, and patent the product so they can exclusively make the health claim for their new product.

"Despite the greater safety of many nutritional medicines, the current legal system fails to provide adequate financial incentives for research to prove that a nutrient has a sufficiently low risk to benefit ratio, and thus favors drugs over nutrients," concluded Dr. Werbach. "For this reason, the benefits of nutritional pharmocotherapy are often poorly validated compared to those of drugs."

For these political reasons, among others, herbal medicines are often viewed as either ineffective or unsafe by the conventional medical establishment. Much of this perception comes from a lack of knowledge. Although it has been clearly proven that the top ten causes of death are directly related to nutrition, less than 40 percent of the medical schools in Canada and United States even offer the minimum hours (only 25) of nutrition training. According to a 1993 article in *SELF* magazine, more than 75 percent of medical schools do not require students to take a single nutrition course. A survey from 15 different medical schools in the United States showed that 65 percent of the graduates were unhappy with the education they received about nutrition.

Unfortunately, the medical establishment is missing out on some very interesting and useful information. There is a large, untapped reservoir of effective medical treatments available. And they're safe.

The Herbal Research Foundation conducted an extensive review on the safety of herbal medicines which was featured in the June 1992 *Food and Drug Law Journal*. According to the article, toxic reactions to herbal products is not a major concern and there is a lack of substantial evidence to indicate otherwise.

"Although numerous herbs growing in the wild can cause significant toxicity, the herbs commonly used in the United States for health purposes are usually safe," explained herbal researcher, author, and lecturer, Michael T. Murray, N.D. "Nonetheless, it is important that you be aware of any possible adverse reactions with herbal product use."

Dr. Murray has written many outstanding books on the subject of natural medicine. I highly recommend his most recent works, *Natural Alternatives to Over-the-Counter and Prescription Drugs* and *The Healing Power of Herbs*. These books will help you determine which treatment plan is best for your particular problem. Both books clearly describe any safety concerns that are present with specific substances. Information about both books is listed in the appendix.

Naturopathic medicine which uses herbs and nutritional supplements enjoys a much better safety record than that of conventional medicine. According to the American Association of Naturopathic Physicians (AANP), "The safety records (of naturopathic doctors) in states with review boards is excellent. Naturopathic physicians can purchase malpractice insurance at extremely low rates. As indicated by such rates, the chance of being injured through malpractice is low."

We will learn that the key to proper naturopathic care is choosing the proper physician. Naturopathic physicians, as well as other natural medicine providers, rely on the scientific evidence that supports the products and treatments they utilize in their practice.

"One of the great myths about natural medicine is that they are not scientific," explained Dr. Murray. "The fact of the matter is, that for most common illnesses there is greater support in the medical literature for a natural approach than there is for drugs or surgery."

**Strong science**

"Scientific studies and observations have not only held up the validity of diet, nutritional supplements, herbal medicines, chiropractic adjustments, and massage, but also some of the more esoteric natural healing treatments including acupuncture, biofeedback, meditation, and homeopathy," explained Dr. Murray, who personally has collected well over 50,000 articles from scientific journals describing the benefits of natural medicine.

Many articles featured in respected peer-reviewed medical journals confirm the benefits of natural medicine products and practices. Because natural medicine is so prevalent in Europe, many of the science originates from foreign professional journals. However, more and more American journals are featuring this information as well.

Over a year ago, I fulfilled a dream—to publish a professional journal for physicians and pharmacists outlining the science of natural medicine. Our journal is called *The American Journal of Natural Medicine* and we are proud to have Dr. Murray as our editor. In the ten issues per year, we review the science regarding natural medicine. (For more information on the journal, refer to this book's appendix.)

An increasing number of conventional medical doctors are taking the time to study the research. We sponsor seminars for healthcare professionals throughout the United States and the response has been very positive. The increase in interest in certain natural medicine disciplines, such as naturopathic, osteopathic, and chiropractic medicine, as well as interest from conventional medical doctors and pharmacists also indicates an increased interest in natural medicine science.

It appears that these healthcare professionals are interested in natural medicine for one or all of these three reasons:

1. Their strong track record.
2. Their low toxicity.
3. The patient demand.

Here are just a few natural medicine topics that have been investigated extensively in the literature:

- Ginkgo biloba for improved blood flow
- Garlic for the heart and entire cardiovascular system
- Glucosamine sulfate for osteoarthritis
- Enteric-coated peppermint oil for irritable bowel syndrome
- Vitamin B6 for carpel tunnel syndrome
- Vitamin E and CoQ10 for the prevention of heart disease
- Calcium and magnesium for bone health
- Folic acid (a B vitamin) to prevent birth defects
- Cranberries for the urinary tract
- Valerian for insomnia
- Feverfew for migraines
- Antioxidants for the prevention of immune system disorders.

And the list goes on and on. The National Institutes of Health Office of Alternative Medicine is using some of its five million dollar budget to study the following:

- Acupuncture for depression.
- Biofeedback for pain control.
- Ayurvedic medicine for Parkinson's disease.
- Prayer for general health.
- Hypnosis to heal broken bones.

Even something as simple as relaxation techniques has been proven scientifically to help prevent and treat very serious illnesses. One study found that when used in conjunction with medical treatment, relaxation therapy reduced the need for medication in 80 percent of study participants with high blood pressure.

Typically, when talking about science and natural medicine, you can expect to hear about the highly publicized Finnish study. The now infamous Finnish study was conducted by the National Cancer Institute (NCI) with $43 million of our hard-earned tax dollars. The NCI said they were trying to find out if beta carotene or vitamin E would help prevent lung cancer. Although the study was riddled with flaws, it received a great deal of media hype. I think it is important to clarify some facts because, unfortunately, the Finnish study is one of the only studies many people refer to regarding vitamins because of the media attention it received.

- The study took place in Finland. Finns have one of the world's highest rates per capita of alcohol consumption among smokers, and it has been well established that alcohol interferes with the utilization of many nutrients, particularly vitamin E and beta carotene.
- Finland is known to have very low levels of the essential mineral, selenium, in the soil, and selenium acts in conjunction with vitamin E in promoting cancer prevention.
- The study group had an average age of 57 and smoked an average of 20 cigarettes per day for almost 37 years straight. Plenty of hard-core, long-term smokers in this group.
- The dosage of both nutrients was much too small for such a high-risk group: only 1/8 to 1/40 the dosage of vitamin E and 1/10 the dosage of beta carotene was used.
- The treatment period was too short, especially for such long-term offenders. Vitamin E and beta carotene are not drugs; they are nutrients that take time to work with the body. Unfortunately, the study participants were given the nutrients at a time when many were already at risk of developing lung cancer, which would then require a therapeutic (high) dose of the nutrients, not a preventive dose.

Given all of these flaws, the study still showed that vitamin E provided protection from prostate cancer. In addition, the researchers confirmed the extremely impressive safety record of these two nutrients. It is unfortunate that the media turned the information around to let people think that these two important vitamins could actually promote the risk of lung cancer. I feel bad for all of the innocent people who threw away their beta carotene and/or vitamin E because of the misinformation connected with this flawed study.

By the way, if you want to help prevent lung cancer, don't smoke! Don't depend on a miracle when it's too late. Make the appropriate changes now and take your vitamins to enhance your chances. It's much safer to rely on your nutritional supplements as prevention rather than choose risky lifestyles and hope your vitamins save you in the final hours. Nutritional supplements are merely weapons in your fight to maintain optimum health—they are not "cure-alls" or magic bullets.

If you are more interested in the science surrounding natural medicine, I suggest you review the many publications, books, and organizations listed in the appendix. You'll find some very exciting information and interesting reading material.

**Chapter summary**

In this chapter we've learned that more people are using natural medicines and visiting alternative practitioners out of a growing frustration with our conventional medical establishment. While safety is a concern for some skeptics, it is one of the main reasons people are turning toward natural medicine. The truth is, natural medicine is safer and often more effective than the conventional medical treatments. While conventional medicine is great at providing crisis care, natural medicine focuses on a more holistic viewpoint, with safety a top priority.

Many natural medicine treatments, products, and services have been studied for centuries and their effectiveness has been confirmed by science. Just as with any medical treatment, you shouldn't participate in any health program without doing your own research up front. The information is there. Search it out and educate yourself. You'll find it will be time well spent.

Now that we've found out that there is a great deal of evidence available validating the safety and science of natural medicine, where do you go from here? How do you get started using natural medicine safely and effectively?

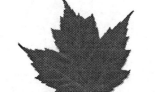

# CHAPTER THREE

## Where Do I Go From Here?

When I first started studying natural medicine, my head was swimming. I began researching nutritional supplements and found the terminology and jargon confusing and over-whelming at times. Fortunately, after I realized that I didn't have to learn everything all at once, I began chipping away at the entire subject, whittling it down into easily digestible pieces. I also found that the more I knew about my body and my needs, the more easily I could understand natural medicine. Your needs and interests should create your learning path. For example, because of my family history of cancer, I have always concentrated on immune function. You may choose to study treatments, services, or products used for cardiovas-cular disease or environmental disorders.

The questions you ask yourself will determine your educational process. What and how you learn begins and ends with you and your needs. Remember, before you can find something, you need to first know what you're looking for.

### Reading the signals

Knowing what you need may seem like a simple concept, but it's not. It wasn't until *after* I got cancer that I truly found out what my body was telling me and how I should respond to the signals—signals that I was ignoring or explaining away.

In July 1994 my sister, Kathi, was operated on for breast cancer.

Although I was trying to be extremely positive, our family history of breast cancer had me concerned about my only sister. We're so close that we even work with each other and have homes next to one another. I began to have "phantom" (fake) pain in my left breast. I quickly disregarded the pain and continued to support my sister the best I could. (As it turns out, it really was fake pain, so when I started to have pain in my abdomen after my mom died, I ignored that, too.)

After consulting with many healthcare professionals including Dr. Charles Simone, Dr. Patrick Quillin, and Dr. Michael Murray, Kathi began taking extra antioxidants (we'll learn more about antioxidants later) and a special product made by Carlson Labs called shark liver oil which contains alkylglycerols. She also had a lumpectomy and radiation therapy. Side effects of radiation include dry, cracking skin, weakness, weight loss, and lethargy. Kathi didn't experience any side effects. She did remarkably well during and after radiation. Her nurses and doctors were calling her their "radiation poster child." Her radiation oncologist told her that if her skin hadn't turned slightly pink, she would have thought they'd forgotten to turn on the machine. Her surgeon has also been shocked at how well she has healed. Of course, Kathi and I know that her nutritional supplement plan has had a huge impact on her recovery. This is a great example of how conventional and natural measures can be used simultaneously for best results. I am very happy to report that Kathi is feeling fantastic!

Within five months after my sister's surgery, my mom became ill. My mom was my first employee at IMPAKT Communications. My sister was my second employee. We were close. Tragically, my mom's cancer was deadly. Within three weeks after I took her to the hospital, she died. The loss was devastating. She was only 58 years old—a vibrant, active individual who, just weeks earlier, was helping us unload boxes of magazines in the warehouse.

During those three weeks, I saw the devastation wrought by a very serious illness. I saw pain and I felt a pain so deep that it's impossible to explain. There is nothing worse than seeing a loved one suffer. But more importantly, I saw courage and was strengthened by my mom's spirituality. She was an incredible woman.

We have an extensive genetic predisposition toward cancer in our family. Both of my grandmothers have had cancer and my grandmother on my mom's side died of the same cancer she had. Three aunts on my mom's side have gotten cancer and two of them have died. One of my dad's sisters also died of breast cancer. Two first cousins are cancer survivors: one breast cancer and the other thyroid cancer. I've met with the University of Wisconsin-Madison genetic counselling center. They believe we either have a cancer cluster or the BRAC1 cancer gene. More research is being conducted. (More on genetic predisposition in Chapter Four.)

As you can see, cancer has had a devastating effect on our family. But I still thought that I was immune. After all, for the past several years I have been doing almost all the right things. I've been taking my vitamins, getting exercise, and watching my diet. But, less than three months after my mom's death, I was operated on for ovarian cancer at age 33.

Just after my sister was diagnosed, I noticed that I started getting pains in my abdomen. I ignored the pain; I thought it wasn't that bad and I had much more important things to think about. After my mom died, the pain worsened. I was depressed about my mom's death and I attributed the pain to the depression. I thought they were psychosomatic (all in my head) because my mom's cancer was in her pancreas, which caused her abdomen to swell. I "blew it off" and kept up the same pace. In hindsight, I was probably a workaholic. I was so used to thinking about work and other people that I never realized that maybe I needed to think about me. I've since learned that if I'm not healthy, I'm no good to anyone else anyway—so, I've made my health a top priority in my life!

Soon, the pain got to the point where it didn't go away. I went to the doctor and he felt the tumor immediately. It was a large mass outside of the ovary pushing my left ovary up and growing down the side of my uterus. I had a complete hysterectomy two days after I turned 33.

I asked my oncologist why I got cancer. Maybe it was a stupid question, but I really wanted to know. He said it was partly because of the stress of my mom's death and our family predisposition. Add to that my "type A" personality and the fact that I always put my needs on the back burner; there's no wonder something happened.

My personal story helps illustrate two important points to remember:

1. You are never immune unless you work on all aspects of your

life and even then there are no absolute guarantees.

2. You need to learn how to read the signals your body sends you.

My body started with brief messages that quickly accelerated to shouts over a loud speaker. And I still ignored the noise until it nearly killed me.

To effectively evaluate what you need you must get to know your body and your mind. It may sound like psychological babble, but you really do need to get in touch with your feelings and learn how to express them with those around you.

I have an incredible support system of family and friends. My cancer battle plan would have been useless without that support and my spiritual commitment. I am fortunate, I had a special angel watching over me during my cancer and I am convinced that's what helped me get through it. There is no question that the death of my mom was much more traumatic than my own cancer. I think I was connecting with her on a whole new level and it was that connection that helped me get through.

I still miss her tremendously, but I talk to her everyday. I've learned to communicate with my mom on a different level. And I think she's still teaching me valuable lessons. She always worried that I worked too hard and that I didn't take care of myself. Today, I believe she knows that I've changed my priorities. I ask myself different questions. My goals are different. And most of all, I've learned how to evaluate my needs more effectively.

## Evaluating your needs

I've been writing about "taking control of your health" and "you're in charge" and "the patient is the customer" for a long time. When my sister and I got cancer, it was time to take my own advice. One thing I've never stopped doing is asking questions. And always remember that the best time to ask yourself questions is before you get to the doctor and before you get sick. Evaluating your needs begins with establishing your health as your number one goal. It has to be at the top of your priority list! Each day, ask yourself this question: What can I do to improve or protect my health today?

Put your healthcare goal in writing along with your other goals. It has been proven that when you write your goals down and review them often, your mind has a better chance at helping you accomplish those goals—and that includes good health. Once you've established that your health is your top priority, it's time to find out just how to accomplish that goal.

Typically, people seek out natural medicine for one of two reasons: the therapeutic benefits when the body is experiencing a crisis; or prevention. You need to determine which category you fit into. Obviously, if you are experiencing a medical emergency (i.e., chest pains, heavy bleeding, trouble breathing, a broken bone, etc.) you need conventional care right away. See your doctor or visit the emergency room of your local hospital.

If you are presently concerned with a specific illness, you need to find out as much as you can about that particular illness. For example, when I found out I had cancer and the doctors were suggesting chemotherapy, I began to research my type of cancer and the types of chemotherapy they were suggesting. My doctors and I later agreed that we would not use chemotherapy because the dangers outweighed any possible benefits. There are lots of great books on the market specifically about natural medicine alternatives for most health conditions. Some excellent books are listed in the appendix of this book. You can also visit your local health food store or book store.

If your goal is to remain healthy and prevent disease, natural medicine provides some wonderful tools you can use to accomplish this goal. Both prevention and therapeutic natural medicine will be discussed further in the next chapter.

As mentioned previously, recognizing specific body functions is important to the success of your natural medicine program. That's why when you are deciding which direction to take, you should begin with a thorough head-to-toe evaluation, paying special attention to a problem or potential problem areas.

Let's give it a try. On a separate piece of paper, answer the following general questions categorized by body function. After each category, jot down your own personal notes as to how you are feeling. You'll be surprised at how much you learn about how your body is functioning.

## Head (central nervous system)
- Do you experience headaches?
- Have you ever experienced a head injury?
- Do you ever have episodes of dizziness?
- Are you experiencing any memory problems?

## Emotional
- Have you been depressed or experienced extended periods of sadness?
- Have you experienced mood swings lately?
- Have you experienced anxiety or nervousness for an extended period of time?
- Do you feel stress or tension on a regular basis (specify daily, weekly, etc.)?

## Endocrine
- Do you have a hypo or hyperthyroid condition?
- Do you have heat or cold intolerances?
- Do you experience excessive thirst or excessive hunger?

## Eyes/Ears/Nose/Sinuses/Throat/Neck
- Do you have impaired vision?
- Do you wear contacts or glasses?
- Do you experience double vision or eye pain?
- Do you experience impaired hearing?
- Do you have ringing in the ears or earaches?
- Do you get nose bleeds?
- Do you experience frequent colds?
- Do you experience stuffiness, hay fever, or sinus problems?
- Do you have swollen glands?
- Are there any lumps in your neck?
- Do you have pain or stiffness in your neck?

## Respiratory
- Do you cough frequently?
- Do you have a history of asthma or bronchitis?
- Have you ever had pneumonia?
- Do you have difficulty breathing or pain upon breathing?
- Any shortness of breath? If so, when?

## Cardiovascular
- Do you have a history of heart disease or high blood pressure?
- Do you have high cholesterol?
- Have you ever experienced chest pain?
- Do you ever experience swelling in the ankles?
- Do you ever experience shortness of breath?

## Gastrointestinal
- Do you have trouble swallowing?
- Do you have frequent bouts of gas, indigestion, and heartburn?
- Do you experience nausea and vomiting?
- How often do you have a bowel movement and has this changed recently?
- Have you ever had hemorrhoids?

## Urinary
- Is there pain upon urination?
- Is there increased frequency of urination, especially at night?
- Do you experience frequent urinary infections?
- Do you experience an inability to hold urine?
- Have you ever had kidney stones?

## Female reproductive
- When did you start your menstrual period?
- How long is your cycle?
- Do you experience breakthrough bleeding between periods?
- Are your cycles regular?

- Do you experience pain during intercourse?
- Do you experience pain during your period?
- Do you experience excessive flow during your period?
- Are you using birth control? If so, what type?
- How many times have you been pregnant (if at all)?
- Have you experienced any miscarriages? If so, how many?
- Have you ever had an abortion?
- Have you ever had difficulty conceiving?
- Have you experienced menopausal symptoms?
- Are you sexually active?
- Have you ever had any sexually transmitted diseases?
- Do you do breast self-exams?
- Have you found any lumps or suspicious sites within your breast?
- Do you experience breast tenderness or pain?

## Male reproductive
- Have you ever had a hernia?
- Have you ever had a mass in your testicle?
- Have you ever experienced testicular pain?
- Are you sexually active?
- Do you experience any sexual difficulties?
- Do you have any symptoms of prostate disorders?
- Do you have venereal disease?
- Do you have any discharge or sores?

## Musculoskeletal
- Do you have any joint pain or stiffness?
- Do you have arthritis? If so, has it been diagnosed as osteoarthritis or rheumatoid arthritis?
- Have you had any broken bones? If so, when and which bones?
- Do you experience any muscle spasms or cramps?
- Do you experience any muscle or bone weakness?

## General

- Have you experienced a weight gain or weight loss of twenty or more pounds within the past year?
- Do you experience easy bleeding or bruising?
- Do you experience fatigue? If so, describe.
- Do you have any skin rashes, eczema, hives, acne, boils, or skin itching?
- Do you have any lumps in any areas of your body that you would consider suspicious or out of the ordinary?

In addition to answering these questions, you should know the following:

- What medications are you presently taking?
- Your family health history in as much detail as possible.
- Your childhood illnesses and health history as much as possible.
- What surgeries and hospital visits have you had?

These evaluation questions were provided by Kevon Arthurs, N.D., of Portland, OR. Dr. Arthurs, like other certified and qualified naturopathic doctors, relies quite heavily on the personal interview with her patients. The evaluation featured previously is the short version. I didn't have room for the longer questionnaire she uses. Dr. Arthurs spends quality time getting to know her patients and their needs. Unfortunately, not all doctors are like Dr. Arthurs. This is why I recommend you take the time to answer these questions before you visit your doctor or start purchasing natural medicine products.

By answering these questions, you will get an idea of what's going on in your body. Any symptoms or problems will surface after you've completed the head-to-toe evaluation. Information may surface that will indicate a visit to a qualified healthcare professional is necessary. If your symptoms are not that serious and you feel self-care is appropriate, take this information into your local health food store or pharmacy and get some direction as to which products would be appropriate for your particular body function concern(s). Or you may discover that you are just as healthy as you thought you were. In that case, you should concentrate on developing a solid prevention program. The advice about diet, exercise, attitude, faith, and nutritional supplements should help.

And believe it or not, this is just the beginning. Remember, health is a very complicated system. To achieve optimal health, you need to continually learn about ways to improve. It's a constant process that includes an honest look at your habits and lifestyle on an ongoing basis. Let's begin by evaluating what you put in your mouth.

## Diet and nutrition

It has been proven that your diet can have a negative or positive impact on your health. Terry Lemerond, president and founder of Enzymatic Therapy, Inc., a nutritional supplement manufacturer, has been studying nutrition for more than 25 years. He writes in his book, *Seven Keys to Vibrant Health*, "The evidence supporting diet's role in chronic degenerative diseases, including heart disease, cancer, stroke, diabetes, and arthritis, is substantial."

There are two basic facts that support the link between diet and disease: (1) a diet rich in plant foods (i.e., whole grains, legumes, fruits, and vegetables) is protective against many diseases while (2) a diet providing a low amount of plant foods can actually cause the development of these diseases.

Think of your body as a highly sophisticated machine. What type of fuel are you putting into your engine? What you eat and drink make up the fuel. Is your diet made up of low-grade fuel or premium quality fuel? What constitutes low-grade or premium fuel anyway?

We've heard about the dangers of a high-fat diet. High-fat foods definitely fall into the low-grade fuel category. They cause your engine to be sluggish and clog important engine parts, like the heart. If you eat a lot of high fat foods, it will be a good idea to reduce your fat intake.

Sugar is another low-grade fuel that can prevent your engine from running efficiently. You may feel a burst of energy after you eat sugary foods, but soon you'll "crash" and experience lower energy levels than before the sugar intake. You should limit your sugar intake. Read labels carefully. You know extra sugar has been added if any one or more of these words appear on the label: sucrose, glucose, maltose, lactose, fructose, corn syrup, or white grape juice concentrate.

According to *Seven Keys to Vibrant Health*, in addition to reducing your fat and sugar intake, you need to limit your salt intake, get plenty of fiber, and eat five or more servings of a combination of fruits and vegetables. Unfortunately, less than ten percent of the American population are presently eating the recommended amount of fruits and vegetables.

Your diet should be made up of whole, unprocessed foods. This type of diet will help you achieve your goal, which is to maintain normal body weight. Obesity is classified as weighing 20 to 30 percent over the average weight for your age, sex, and height. It has been estimated that more than 34 million Americans are overweight. Obesity is associated with an increased risk for many chronic, serious illnesses. That's why it is so important to maintain an ideal body weight.

It's not an easy task as we are bombarded with fast food and enticing advertising for foods that are not good for us. Here's a sad statistic: In 1993, while the National Cancer Institute spent $400,000 on its "5-A-Day for Better Health" program to encourage people to eat more fruits and vegetables, Kellogg spent $32 million just to advertise its sugar leyden Frosted Flakes cereal, according to *Nutrition Action* 1994 and *U.S. News and World Report* 1994. Although it may not be easy, eating properly is necessary if you want to maintain optimum health or treat illness.

And just a quick word about dieting—don't! Take it from someone who has tried many diets, until you decide to make a lifestyle change, chances are you will not have long-term success on a short-term diet. Make a commitment to eat more nutritious, healthful foods and you'll reach your normal weight sooner than you expect.

---

According to a recent Harris poll, nearly three out of four Americans are overweight. The national survey found that 79 percent of men and 64 percent of women are too fat. The poll found that generally the proportion of overweight people increased with age. Earlier studies have also confirmed that 60 percent of the American public can be classified as sedentary, which indicates that their key activity is sitting.

—*PT Bulletin*, March 1995

# Weight Chart

The following provides an acceptable weight range that coincides with optimum health. An additional thirty pounds over the highest point of the weight range below means you would be categorized as obese and are at higher risk of developing certain illnesses like heart disease and cancer.

| Height | Men | Women |
|---|---|---|
| 5'0" | | 96-125 |
| 5'1" | | 99-128 |
| 5'2" | 112-141 | 102-131 |
| 5'3" | 115-144 | 105-134 |
| 5'4" | 118-148 | 108-138 |
| 5'5" | 121-152 | 111-142 |
| 5'6" | 124-156 | 114-146 |
| 5'7" | 128-161 | 118-150 |
| 5'8" | 132-166 | 122-154 |
| 5'9" | 136-170 | 126-158 |
| 5'10" | 140-174 | 130-163 |
| 5'11" | 144-179 | 134-168 |
| 6'0" | 148-184 | 138-173 |
| 6'1" | 152-189 | |
| 6'2" | 156-194 | |
| 6'3" | 160-199 | |
| 6'4" | 164-204 | |

Remember, gradual weight loss is much healthier than quick changes in weight. Changes in body fat should take place on a slow steady basis.

**Exercise regularly**

There are three words to remember when it comes to maintaining or achieving optimum health: exercise, exercise, exercise. The benefits of exercise on the body as well as the mind cannot be overstated.

We are often cautioned to check with our doctor before starting an exercise program; unfortunately, we are rarely cautioned about the dangers of *not* starting an exercise program. There is no doubt that the more active you are the better chance you will have at fending off illness and gaining good health.

A regular exercise program will benefit your entire body. It will also help you maintain normal body weight. Exercise increases muscle and muscle tissue is the primary user of calories in the body. So, it follows that the more muscle you have, the more fat you will burn as energy and the more weight you will lose.

An added benefit of exercise is its effect on your mind as well as your body. Regular exercise has been shown to release tensions, help you deal with stress, reduce depressions, and enhance your self image.

Experts agree that it takes a minimum of twenty minutes, three to five times per week to get the benefits of exercise. Your exercise program should include activities to improve cardiovascular endurance, muscle strength and flexibility.

It is important to select activities you will enjoy. Exercise should be fun, not a chore. Exercise also doesn't have to mean spandex and pumping iron. Although you should incorporate some type of strengthening activities into your regimen, mere walking can provide you with an excellent workout and doesn't require special clothing or equipment, except for good walking shoes.

If you make physical activity a regular part of your health program, you will reap the benefits. Stay motivated by setting exercise goals and

---

Regular exercise has been shown to be an effective treatment of, among other things, glaucoma. In addition, regular exercise or the involvement in moderate to heavy sports activities has been shown to protect against Parkinson's disease.
—*Archives of Opthamology* 1991
   *Archives of Neurology* 1992                              ✌

varying your routine. Remember, your body was meant to move. Keep it active and it will keep you healthy.

By the way, if you are out of shape or have had past health problems, you should consult with your physician before beginning your exercise program.

There's no better time to start exercising than today. Make the commitment—you'll be glad you did.

### Attitude adjustment

Science has confirmed what natural medicine practitioners have known for decades: Your thoughts and emotions have a big impact on your health!

Stress-related symptoms continue to account for 70 percent of all physician office visits, according to a leading research and educational institute in northern California. According to the Institute of HeartMath (IHM), $200 billion each year is spent by businesses throughout the United States on stress and stress-related illnesses. In addition, estimates show that at least 40 percent of employee turnover is due to stress, according to *California Business* (April 1993).

More importantly, the link between stress and disease has been firmly established. As reported by *California Business*, "In a landmark 20-year study conducted at the University of London, researchers found that negative reactions to stress were the single most dangerous risk factor for cancer and heart disease—worse than smoking or high cholesterol foods."

Recognizing the dramatic effects stress has on people is only half the battle—the easy part. Finding ways to effectively cope with stress and anxiety seems to be the real challenge.

Could it be that a simple attitude adjustment upon recognizing stressful feelings such as frustration, anger, and anxiety will actually not only help the situation, but get us back on the road to a healthier future? That seems to be the conclusion of recent research being released by the IHM—if we can control our thoughts and emotions we can improve our cardiovascular and overall health.

"At the root of personal and professional stress lies perception. It is how we perceive and react to the stressful events in our day that determines how much stress we carry with us, and how much our minds, bodies and hearts are taxed," according to IHM's Director of Corporate

Programs, Bruce Cryer.

The IHM, which is a nonprofit research organization, has recently developed a program to improve the health and effectiveness of individuals and organizations. The technique, which is being utilized nationally by many large corporations and all four branches of the United States military, is called Freeze-Frame.

"Freeze-Frame allows us to temporarily disengage from our current perception that is causing the internal turmoil, and open a window of opportunity to see more options and then take efficient and effective action," explains Cryer.

The goal of Freeze-Frame and true stress control is to prevent stressful reactivity or at least disengage from one's emotions and get to neutral in the moment, while it is occurring. One of the benefits is protecting the body's immune system while fending off the negative effects of stress. IHM has discovered that stress and the many emotions associated with stress (i.e. anger, frustration, anxiety) actually deplete a key immune system antibody known as IgA. "This antibody, more than any other, is the body's first line of defense against bacteria," explained Cryer.

According to the *Employee Health & Fitness* newsletter, in one study involving 20 HeartMath employees, "a single, five-minute episode of anger produced a brief increase in IgA. Then, it dropped steadily to one-half its previous level, and seven hours later it still had not returned to normal. Conversely, a five-minute period of caring and compassion caused a dramatic increase in IgA, boosting the immune system."

Presently, there is a case study evaluating the Freeze-Frame technique taking place at Southamptom University Medical School in England involving 600 patients with high blood pressure. "In the field of stress management...the techniques taught by the Institute of HeartMath are the cutting edge," explained Dr. Alan Watkins, a research fellow at Southamptom University. "Their practice bestows confidence that you can manage any situation whether personal or professional."

Exciting information continues to be released by the IHM. Their research has clearly shown that emotions such as caring, compassion, and appreciation can increase your ability to fight disease, while anger actually lowers your resistance levels. According to Professor Jerry

Ainsworth of Southern Connecticut State University, love is one of those emotions that can actually improve your health. "Get and give plenty of love," recommends Ainsworth, who teaches a course at the University called Love and Health.

Research has shown that the very organ most affected by stress and emotional distress may, in fact, hold the key to successful health as well—the heart. "When people make a sincere effort to have more caring attitudes toward other people, it really does boost the body's immune system. A Harvard study determined that in 1988 and we've confirmed it many times since then," explained Cryer.

Using the heart to protect the heart—it's a concept that the IHM says works more effectively than any other stress management technique ever introduced. No more "grinning and bearing it"—no more "burning out"—and no more "hangin' on 'til Friday." It's time to take control of your emotions and take charge! It's time for an attitude adjustment.

Without question, the mind/body connection is one of the most important relationships we have to protect our health. Our thoughts and emotions and how we deal with those thoughts and emotions will contribute, either negatively or positively to our overall health and well-being. How we respond to people and how they respond to us will also have critical health implications. So, the next time you want to "snap" at your neighbor, think of your health and find something nice to say!

### Faith: The forgotten factor in healthcare

For people who are spiritual, you don't need to say much about the importance of faith because they've already experienced the power. Today, science is recognizing the strong relationship between spirituality and our health and the health of our loved ones.

Although "the faith factor" has rarely been studied under strict scientific circumstances, the times that it has been studied have proven it is a very positive part of any health program. As reported in the *American Journal of Natural Medicine* (May 1995), David Larson, M.D. revealed that the findings in two psychiatry journals during 12 years showed religious commitment measures of ceremony, social support, prayer, and relationship with God to be beneficial 92 percent of the time. What is even more impressive, is that there was a study showing that those who were prayed for—and didn't know they were being prayed for—had better health results than those people who were not being prayed for.

Dr. Larson explained that studies have shown prayer and faith will actually help prevent high blood pressure. In one study, men aged 55 or older who ranked religion as very important had diastolic blood pressure six millimeters lower than those who rated religion as somewhat or not important. "Not only do the religiously committed have a greater chance to live longer, but they are more satisfied with their life," concluded Dr. Larson.

I was fortunate to have a very positive religious role model to follow. My mom was very religious. During the last weeks of her life, her spirituality helped her prepare for what was to come. She was at peace and that helped us cope with the devastating loss. One night, toward the end, she woke me in the middle of the night to tell me that I didn't need to worry about her. She said, "He's already here with me. He holds me at night and he said he'll walk with me the entire way."

No, faith did not save my mom's life—it gave her a new life. I pray to her every night. I suggest that some type of spiritual connection is necessary for true healing and optimum health to take place.

As always, we need to look at everything that is available to us to help us in our search for superior health and a fulfilling life. Faith, prayer, spirituality—they all add up to another option that we may want to take advantage of.

## Nutritional supplements

It wasn't too long ago when some people were afraid to go inside a health food store. What would they find? After all, we all knew that these stores were filled with granola-eating, voodoo-practicing hippies, right? Wrong! I've been shopping in our local health food store for about six years now and I have had the real pleasure of visiting countless health food stores throughout the United States. As a matter of fact, whenever I travel, I try and visit the local health food store.

What I've found is the most caring group of individuals I have ever met in an industry. Health food store owners, managers and employees are often motivated by their own success story. Chances are, they got involved in the natural health industry because they wanted to "spread the word." For the most part, their motives are pure and their knowledge is extensive.

Let's take my local health food store as an example. Bay Natural Foods is managed by Sue Kranick. Sue has been with Bay Natural Foods since she was a teenager. Her knowledge of nutritional supplements and natural medicine is impressive. I rely heavily on Sue to provide me with the latest information on natural medicine and to help guide me on my path to good health. You should do the same. Of course, you won't be able to rely on Sue (unless you live in Green Bay, WI), but you probably have a "Sue" in one of your local health food stores. If you haven't already, visit your local health food store. You will be amazed at all the great items you can find there. If you don't have a health food store in your neighborhood, you'll have to get your information from books, magazines, and possibly a natural healthcare provider.

Nutritional supplements are a key item in all health food stores. The selection is extensive and unfortunately can be confusing. Here are some quick facts about nutritional supplements that might help to clear things up.

- Nutritional supplements are vitamins, minerals, herbal extracts, amino acids, glandular extracts or a combination of any of these designed to support specific body functions or contribute to your overall well-being (the "tonic" effect).
- Nutritional supplements are not drugs and they are not food items. They are dietary supplements and they are regulated as dietary supplements.
- Just because something is "natural" does not make it effective or safe.

Reading the label is important when you buy nutritional supplements. Never buy any product that does not clearly state what's in it and how much of the particular ingredient(s) are in it.

Let's use the example of a product on the market called Formula One, which is a multi-level marketing product that is not sold in health food stores. I know many people who have gotten excellent results from the product; however, after looking at the label when the product first hit the market, I immediately noticed that the milligram amounts were not listed. The product simply stated the ingredients but did not tell me how much of each ingredient was in each capsule. This worries me because there is no way of knowing *exactly* what you are putting into your body.

In addition to reading the label, here are the other guidelines I use when I am purchasing a nutritional supplement:

- If I feel uneasy about anything regarding the product I am considering, I don't take it.
- I always clarify how much I should be taking and ask lots of questions about the product. That's why I shop in a health food store and not at a supermarket—the customer support is excellent.
- I typically buy products with some type of guarantee. That's why I use a lot of Enzymatic Therapy products. Enzymatic Therapy has the best guarantee in the natural health industry. If I use the whole bottle but don't get any results I can take it back and get a full refund. This type of money back guarantee shows me that the manufacturer has a great deal of faith in his/her products, and I like that.
- I only use herbal products that are standardized. Standardization is a scientific process that ensures quality and consistency among herbal products. An herb usually has an active component that makes it effective. Each plant is unique and does not contain the same amount of active components. When an herb is standardized for that specific component you know that each capsule or tablet has that same amount of active component. Dr. Michael Murray was extremely instrumental in getting the standardization process to the United States market. Without standardization, one capsule could have lots of activity while another capsule, in the same bottle, could have no activity. The herbs in the Formula One product were not standardized when I last looked at the label. It's possible that they now include standardized herbs in their product.

Here are some examples of popular herbs that are standardized for active components:

- European bilberry—Used for eye health, bilberry extracts should be standardized to contain 25 percent anthocyanidins with a standard dose of 80 to 160 mg three times daily.
- Ginkgo biloba—For blood flow and circulation, ginkgo contains ginkgoheterosides and should contain a standardized amount of 25 percent at a dose of 40 mg three times daily.
- Kava—Used as anti-anxiety formula, kava extract should be standardized for its kavalactone content at 30 percent.

- Valerian—As a mild sedative and sleep aid, valerian extract should be standardized to contain 0.8 percent valeric acid at a dose of 150 to 300 mg of the extract.

The list goes on. Remember, when buying an herbal supplement, make sure the label "spells out" just what the active component is and how much of the standardized amount is in each product. Remember, without standardization, there are no guarantees as to what or how much each capsule or tablet contains.

When you start reading more about natural medicine, you will become very good at distinguishing an inferior product from a superior one. There's no doubt that getting the right product can make all the difference in the world. Let me give you an example.

I purchase a product called Super Saw Palmetto extract for my dad. The product is designed to help prevent and alleviate enlarged prostate. It has been shown that nearly 60 percent of men from age 40 to 59 have an enlarged prostate. I've read the research on enlarged prostate and how this herb helps. There are lots of Saw palmetto extract products on the market, so how did I choose the right one? I read the label and matched the label with the studies that have been done.

The dosage of the Enzymatic Therapy Super Saw Palmetto extract that I buy for my dad is 160 milligrams standardized to contain 85 to 95 percent fatty acids and sterols, which is identical to the dosage used in the clinical studies. Sitting right next to the Super Saw Palmetto extract is another product that contains 500 mg of Saw palmetto extract at one-half the cost of the product I buy. So, why don't I buy that product? Because in this case, the milligram amount is not the only determining factor. I know that if 500 mg of the extract is not standardized to contain the 85 to 95 percent fatty acids and sterols, it won't work for my dad. Rather than saving money, I would be throwing my money away.

Still another example is St. John's wort. After my mom died, I was experiencing depression. I had read about the studies on St. John's wort for mild to moderate depression, and I decided to give it a try. It has helped my depression and I remain on the product today. The product I use is standardized to contain 0.3 percent hypericin (the active component) and contains 300 mg of the extract per capsule. Other products that are not standardized in this way may simply have ground up St. John's wort leaves in the capsule and have absolutely no therapeutic value. If I were to buy any of these other products, I may have saved money in the short term, but I would not have been helped, resulting in frustration and valuable time and money wasted.

This helps to illustrate that you must use care when purchasing nutritional supplements. The people in your health food store will be a big help. Learn to rely on them; if not for their advice, then for the informational literature they can provide to you. Also, let your body be your judge. If you're feeling better, stick with the product. If you're not feeling better after a reasonable time period (some products may take up to three months before you see results), try something else.

**Chapter summary**

It is absolutely critical that you recognize your body signals and learn how to effectively evaluate your needs. Set some health goals and do a head-to-toe inventory before using natural medicine or seeing a natural medicine provider to get an idea of your individual needs.

Pay close attention to your diet. What you eat and drink plays a huge part in your health. Just as diet is extremely important, so is exercise. Exercise regularly for at least twenty minutes three times a week.

Use caution when purchasing nutritional supplements and become an active label reader. Get as much information about a particular product before taking it and ask if the product is guaranteed. Remember, cheaper does not always mean you will save money in the long run and it definitely doesn't mean you're getting the best product. When it comes to your health, you'll find that nutritional supplements are an important investment.

Now let's take a closer look at how to use natural medicine and how to incorporate it into your health regimen.

## Quick Reference Guide

Although the following nutrients and herbs serve a variety of important purposes, here is a quick look at some of the main applications.

| Nutrient/Herb | Condition/Usage |
| --- | --- |
| Vitamin A | enhanced immune function |
| Vitamin C | enhanced immune function |
| Vitamin E | immune and cardiovascular system |
| B-Vitamins | stress/central nervous system |
| Folic acid | prevention of birth defects |
| Zinc | antioxidant/male reproductive system |
| Calcium | bone health/osteoporosis prevention |
| Magnesium | bone health/cardiovascular health |
| Potassium | cardiovascular |
| Glucosamine sulfate | osteoarthritis |
| L-Tryptophan | depression and anxiety |
| Hypericin | antihistamine |
| Enzymes | proper digestion |
| Ginkgo | brain function/improved blood flow |
| Silymarin | liver disorders/detoxification |
| Echinacea | immune system disorders |
| Saw palmetto | enlarged prostate/prostate health |
| Bilberry extract | eye disorders/eye health |
| Gugulipids | lowers cholesterol |
| Curcumin | reduces inflammation |
| St. John's wort | depression |
| Valerian | insomnia |
| Grape seed extract | antioxidant/vascular disorders |
| Melissa extract (topical) | cold sores and Herpes simplex |
| Garlic | immune system/cardiovascular |
| Ginseng | overall well-being/energy |
| Hawthorn extract | cardiovascular health |
| Kava extract | anxiety |
| Peppermint extract | irritable bowel syndrome |

# CHAPTER FOUR

## How Do I Use
## Natural Medicine?

T aking advantage of the options that are best for you is critical to your healthcare success. But before we can learn how to use natural medicine, we must first review the services, treatments, and products that are available (definitions are provided in chapter one):

- acupuncture
- ayurvedic medicine
- biofeedback
- body work (massage, reiki, rolfing, etc.)
- chelation therapy
- chiropractic care
- comprehensive patient questionnaire
- detoxification therapy
- diagnostic tests
- glandular therapy
- guided imagery
- herbal medicines
- homeopathy
- hydrotherapy
- hypnotherapy
- nutritional and psychological counselling
- nutritional supplements

Although this is not a complete listing of all the natural medicine services available to you, these are the main ones that you will be exposed to during your search for information about natural medicine alternatives. These services, treatments, and products should provide you with a great starting point.

As mentioned previously, people usually search out alternative healthcare options for one of two reasons: To prevent illness or to help with a specific condition or concern.

## Prevention

It is much better emotionally, physically, and financially, to try to prevent illness rather than get rid of a disease after it takes hold. Unfortunately, serious illnesses run rampant in our society.

Jan McBarron, M.D., reminds us of some very scary health facts in her book *Flavor Without Fat*:

- Every minute, a person suffers a heart attack.
- Every year, between 600,000 and 800,000 people die of a heart attack.
- Every year, 70,000 people are diagnosed with colon cancer and five years later, one-half of them are dead.
- Every 13 minutes, another woman dies of breast cancer (one out of every 10 women will develop breast cancer), which is the same rate as in 1950.
- More than 25,000 men die of prostate cancer each year.

Researchers are learning what natural medicine practitioners knew decades ago: Our nutritional status is a key contributor to our health. Unfortunately, we are a country that is overfed and undernourished. An introduction to the American diet begins with sugar and ends with fat. Government statistics from 1993 showed that the typical American diet is made up of 40 to 60 percent fat. Over the past several decades, fat consumption has increased by more than 30 percent and sugar consumption has jumped up over 50 percent.

Here are the *1992 Top Ten Almanac* top ten brands purchased in grocery stores (ranked by dollar volume):

- cigarettes (number 1 and 10)
- soda pop (number 2, 3, and 5)
- beer (number 7)
- coffee (number 9)

Fast foods, deep-fried foods, processed foods, white flour, and sweets represent a large portion of the American diet—empty calories lacking nutritional value. If your top ten grocery item list looks like the list above, you are a prime candidate for illness and you need to make some serious changes.

The most effective prevention program begins with lifestyle factors you can control. As mentioned in Chapter Three, health starts with you and the things you do. Eating a healthful diet, avoiding fat and nutritionally barren foods, will get you on your way to better health, more energy, and a happier life. In addition to paying close attention to your diet, here are other lifestyle factors you must deal with if you are really interested in preventing illness:

- If you smoke, quit!
- If you drink alcohol, do it in moderation, or not at all.
- Get regular exercise and physical activity.
- Find quality time to relax and enjoy life.
- Laugh a lot and laugh regularly.
- Be good to others and give of yourself.
- Be optimistic and think positively.
- Practice some form of spirituality.

Volumes have been written on how your attitude affects your health. Scientific studies and very solid research support the fact that positive, optimistic people who are spiritual and supported spiritually by friends and family are more likely to deal successfully with serious illness. (For more on emotional health, refer to "Attitude Adjustment" in Chapter Three.)

When I was told I had cancer, my friends and family rallied around me. The best medicine I was given didn't come from my doctor or wasn't in any of my vitamin bottles; it came from family and friends. Many readers wrote to me and called the office to tell me they were praying for me or thinking about me and my family. These people were virtually strangers, but they found the time to let me know that they cared. That's pretty powerful. If we could bottle that caring energy and give it to all of those suffering in this world, we'd have no more suffering.

Taking a look at your support system and the types of people you surround yourself with is one important first step in taking control of your health. You need to be in charge of your prevention program. We've all heard that "an ounce of prevention is worth a pound of cure." The reason we've all heard that so much is that it's true! Take control as much as you can before disease strikes. Understand, however, that there are no guarantees in life.

## A word about other causes

Our environment can have a big impact on our health. We've learned in previous chapters that environmental stresses can wreak havoc on our bodies. Pollution, poor drinking water, and other toxins in the environment around us can actually contribute to illnesses. The paper mills and nuclear power plants definitely have a negative impact on our environment. Whether or not these environmental toxins actually cause disease is still debatable; however, there is plenty of evidence that says they contribute to disease.

Breast cancer provides us with a prime example of a disease that has been linked to environmental toxins. In an eye-opening article featured in the *International Journal of Health Services* (Vol. 24, No. 1, 1994), Samuel Epstein, M.D. revealed, "For over three decades, evidence has accumulated relating avoidable exposures to environmental and occupational carcinogens to the escalating incidence of breast cancer in the United States and other major industrialized nations."

Dr. Epstein discovered that the scientifically substantiated connection between environmental toxins and breast cancer has been completely ignored by the National Cancer Institute and the American Cancer Society despite expenditures of more than one billion dollars on breast cancer research. "A variety of occupational exposures has been incriminated as risk factors for breast cancer," concluded Dr. Epstein. Among them, pesticides, chlorinated solvents, hair dyes, and estrogens. And breast cancer is just one example of the connection between environmental toxins and illness.

In addition to our environment, our genetic makeup can give us a particular tendency for specific conditions.

One of the biggest mistakes we make when we do get sick, especially if we were trying so hard to stay healthy, is to place blame. Oftentimes we blame ourselves, which is unproductive and unhealthy. When I got cancer, I was actually ashamed. Here I was, the publisher of three national health magazines, and I got cancer. Today, I feel compelled to share what I have learned so it may help other people.

As mentioned previously, I have a genetic predisposition toward cancer. The women in our family, including my extended family of cousins, aunts, and nieces, have either the BRAC1 breast cancer/ovarian cancer gene, or we have a cancer cluster. Considering that my mom and her mom both died of pancreatic cancer, there is more of a chance that we have a cancer cluster, which is a predisposition toward a variety of cancers.

It is very important to clarify that a predisposition toward a specific condition does not mean you will get that condition. It simply means that you have a better chance of getting that disease than someone else who does not have a predisposition. Just as with cancer, the same is true for heart disease and other illnesses. If you have a family history of heart disease, you need to take extra precautions to prevent a heart attack.

So, why did I get cancer? The same reason other people get cancer—a combination of factors, which included stress. I forgot about a very important element of a comprehensive prevention program:

• Stress Reduction. Prior to my illness, I was a workaholic. Instead of trying to reduce the stress in my life, I just continued to "stuff" it. As a publisher, I deal with deadlines all the time; however, that's not the stress that can cause illness. If your workday is managed properly and efficient systems are in place, your work should not get stressful enough to affect your health. My work was affecting my health because I never let it go. I concentrated on my company around the clock with very little time for myself or for relaxation. In addition, the stress of my sister and my mom's illnesses was deeply stressful. I have learned to deal with stress much better. Here are my recommendations for having a less stressful existence (and remember, not all stress is bad—it's the stress that negatively affects your health that you have to worry about):

1. Take time to rest and relax away from work.
2. Do things you enjoy and have fun!
3. Do things for yourself. (For example, I try to get a massage every other week.)

Since my illness, I have restructured my goals. I have different priorities. I'm less serious and more relaxed than ever before.

Presently, I am at more than a 50 percent risk of developing breast cancer because of my ovarian cancer and the fact that I now must take estrogen. But, I don't let my genetic predisposition or this new cancer risk scare me. I am optimistic and I am in control.

### Nutritional supplements

One way I continue to stay in control of my health is with nutritional supplements. As we learned earlier, nutritional supplements (often called vitamins) are products that contain one or more vitamin, mineral, herb, amino acid, or glandular ingredient. Nutritional supplements can be very important tools to help prevent or treat illness.

One of the best ways to purchase nutritional supplements is to use products for specific body functions. Here are some prime examples:

**The immune system.** Antioxidant nutrients (vitamins C and E, beta carotene, zinc, and selenium) are very important in stimulating proper immune function. An antioxidant is a compound that prevents free-radical damage. Free radicals are toxins that can destroy your immune system. If the immune system is well nourished with antioxidants it has a better chance of keeping your body healthy. When Dr. Linus Pauling said vitamin C could cure the common cold or help prevent cancer, he was laughed out of many prestigious universities. But Dr. Pauling got the last laugh when all of the scientific studies confirmed his earlier statements.

In addition to antioxidants, there are other ways to stimulate the immune system. Many herbs, for example, have been shown to enhance immunity even better than the highly touted antioxidant nutrients like vitamins C and E. Herbs such as echinacea, procyanodolic flavonoids from grape seeds (also known as PCOs), and garlic are great for the immune system. I take a product that contains many of the nutrients and herbs for the immune system. It's called CPS (Cellular Protection System) by Enzymatic Therapy. This product is known as a formulation (one or more important ingredients). The reason I chose this product is because it contains enough of the nutrients listed. I'm always wary of products that have very small milligram amounts. We'll talk more about this under the section, "RDAs not enough." In addition to CPS, I take a liquid echinacea product, EchinaFresh, to bolster my immune system. The liquid form is more quickly and easily absorbed.

There is also a glandular product that can be used to stimulate the immune system—thymus extract. Particularly useful with individuals suffering from the hepatitis virus, thymus extracts nourish the thymus gland in the body, which is the master gland of the immune system.

In our late twenties, our thymus gland begins to weaken. Researchers speculate that if you keep the thymus gland stimulated, you will be better able to fend off certain immune-compromising illnesses. In Europe, thymus extract is a very popular prescription drug. I recommend a product called ThymuPlex or Thymulus because these products contain the exact polypeptide fractions from the thymus extract that was used in the studies.

I had the pleasure of interviewing the famous country singer Naomi Judd. As you may know, Hepatitis C has caused Naomi to discontinue her career. She is presently in remission and attributes her good health to prayer, positive thinking, support from family and friends, and thymus extract. She's convinced that the thymus extract has made a world of difference in her life. When I was interviewing her, Naomi was full of energy and spunk. It was truly difficult to tell that she has such a serious, life-threatening illness. Hepatitis C is incurable.

**Joints and bone structure.** The immune system is always such a great place to start when it comes to prevention; however, when I'm giving examples of nutritional supplements that really make a difference, I have to mention osteoporosis and arthritis. Bone strength, especially for women who have a family history of osteoporosis, is so important. I take a product called OsteoPrime that was developed by two of the most highly respected medical professionals in the natural health industry, Alan Gaby, M.D., and Jonathan Wright, M.D. I recommend that women begin taking OsteoPrime in their early twenties.

For arthritis, there is a natural compound that has really taken the industry by storm. The studies on the effectiveness of glucosamine sulfate on osteoarthritis are very impressive. Dr. Michael Murray, who always seems to be on the cutting edge of natural health research, was instrumental in bringing this product and information to the American marketplace. I have talked with many individuals who have found a tremendous benefit from the glucosamine sulfate product they are taking. My dad and my aunt take a product called ArMax, which contains 500 mg of the glucosamine sulfate. What I like about this product is that it contains so many other great ingredients for bone health, including calcium, magnesium, and boron.

Although these are just a few examples, the concept is that after you identify which areas of the body need support, there are specific product formulations that can help improve those body functions. Supplements that help nourish weakened body systems or help maintain good overall health are available. You can get the specific products that I have mentioned at your local health food store. There are toll-free numbers in the appendix that will help you find a store in your area that carries the products.

One final note: Nutritional supplements are not magic bullets or should not be considered the only part of your healthcare program—they are just one important piece of the puzzle. Use them wisely and they will provide you with great benefit.

## RDAs are not enough

There is startling evidence to suggest that nutritional deficiencies are very common in the United States today. We are living in a nation that is overfed and undernourished. Many studies now suggest that nutritional deficiencies are much more common than ever expected.

According to a 1987 report in the *Archives of Internal Medicine*, "Between 25 and 50 percent of patients admitted to an acute medical service are malnourished. Physicians are often unaware which patients are admitted at nutritional risk and make no attempt to arrest further nutritional decline until a dramatic deterioration has occurred."

In addition to people who are ill, there are many other groups that are at risk of having nutritional deficiencies. According to Melvyn R. Werbach, M.D. these groups include but are not limited to:

- adolescents
- cigarette smokers
- diabetics
- prescription drug users
- dieters seeking weight loss
- moderate to heavy consumers of alcohol
- women who are pregnant, lactating, or on oral contraceptives

"While many people fall into more than one group, it is clear that a substantial proportion of the population is at increased risk of malnutrition," concludes Dr. Werbach.

Women, the elderly, teenagers, and people who are ill are most at risk of having one or more nutritional deficiencies. In addition to these groups, it is estimated that only about nine percent of adults manage to consumer the five servings of fruits and vegetables daily recommended by the United States dietary guidelines. In a 1989 survey by the United States Department of Agriculture, of 21,500 people surveyed, not one of them consumed 100 percent of the Recommended Dietary Allowance (RDA) for ten of the essential nutrients in a three-day period.

According to a 1991 article featured in *Health Counselor,* Americans are typically deficient in these essential nutrients:
- 90 percent are deficient in chromium
- 80 percent in vitamin B6
- 75 percent in magnesium
- 68 percent in calcium
- 57 percent in iron
- 50 percent in vitamin A
- 45 percent in vitamin B1
- 41 percent in vitamin C
- 34 percent in vitamin B2 and B12
- 33 percent in niacin

In one of the richest countries in the world, the United States, evidence tells us that malnutrition is a key problem that can result in disease and death. Meticulously monitoring the American diet, getting plenty of exercise, and using supplements when necessary may be the best plan of attack in our fight against malnutrition. And one aspect has become quite clear—the RDAs are not proper indicators of nutritional value in our foods.

Did you know that the RDAs for specific nutrients was developed more than 50 years ago? Long before food processing, increased sugar and fat consumption, and countless prescription and over-the-counter medications, the RDAs were established to tell people how much of a particular nutrient they needed to avoid the corresponding nutrient disease. For example, the RDA for vitamin C was established so people would not die from scurvy. However, Dr. Linus Pauling insisted that these nutrients need to be taken in much higher dosages to obtain optimal health, not just prevent disease. The RDAs are just not high enough.

Dr. Pauling, who was a brilliant man and the only person to win two unshared Nobel Prizes, concluded that 100 times the RDA for vitamin C is necessary for optimum health. Dr. Pauling, who lived to be 93 years old, was at one point taking 18 grams of vitamin C daily (that's 18,000 milligrams!). He later discovered that vitamin C not only helped stimulate the immune system, it helped prevent heart disease, as well.

Countless researchers and prestigious organizations including the United States Department of Agriculture's Human Nutrition Research Center now agree that the RDAs do not optimize body function and help prevent chronic disease. A higher quantity of a variety of nutrients is required to help prevent degenerative diseases. A great example of this is folic acid. Despite literally decades of hard science confirming that folic acid will prevent neural tube defects in infants (such as spina bifida), it wasn't until just recently that the United States Public Health Service began advising all women of childbearing age to take 400 micrograms of folic acid. The government is virtually telling women to disregard the RDA and that it is far too low to help prevent illness to their children. Unfortunately, the government knew about this years earlier. Countless lives could have been saved and emotional suffering prevented!

Here are just some of the key activities that can rob your body of important nutrients and why supplementing the diet may be necessary:
- food processing
- sugar and fat consumption
- consumption of alcohol
- smoking
- taking medications
- dieting/calorie counting
- varying individual needs (history of illness, etc.)
- stress
- food allergies
- poor digestion

Only those who live a very pure and uneventful life are not exposed to any of the above. Depending on the degree, nutritional supplementation may be necessary. At a bare minimum, you should be taking a very comprehensive multi-vitamin formula. Here's the label of the multi-vitamin/mineral formula I take. Compare it to yours and make sure it stands up to the challenge. By the way, the following label is from a multiple especially designed for women and it's called Doctor's Choice for Women developed by respected researcher Dr. Michael Murray. Fortunately, Dr. Murray also designed a formula for men called Doctor's Choice for Men.

Each three tablets contain (I take three tablets daily):

| Essential Vitamins and Minerals: | | percent RDA |
|---|---|---|
| Vitamin A (Beta carotene) | 15,000 IU | 300 |
| Vitamin A (Retinol) | 2,500 IU | 50 |
| Vitamin E | 200 IU | 667 |
| Vitamin D | 100 IU | 25 |
| Calcium | 400 mg | 40 |
| Vitamin C | 300 mg | 500 |
| Magnesium | 300 mg | 75 |
| Potassium | 99 mg | ** |
| Vitamin B | 690 mg | 4,500 |
| Niacin/Niacinamide | 90 mg | 450 |
| Thiamine (Vitamin B1) | 60 mg | 4,000 |
| Riboflavin (Vitamin B2) | 60 mg | 3,529 |
| Pantothenic acid | 30 mg | 300 |
| Zinc | 20 mg | 133 |
| Iron | 18 mg | 100 |
| Manganese | 5 mg | ** |
| Vitamin B | 65 mg | 250 |
| Copper | 1 mg | 50 |
| Folic acid | 800 mcg | 200 |
| Vitamin B1 | 2800 mcg | 13,333 |
| Biotin | 600 mcg | 200 |
| Iodine (Kelp) | 300 mcg | 200 |
| Chromium Polynicotinate | 200 mcg | ** |
| Selenium | 200 mcg | ** |
| Vitamin K | 60 mcg | ** |
| Molybdenum | 25 mcg | ** |

(**No RDA has been established for this nutrient)

<u>Other Ingredients:</u>

| | |
|---|---|
| Flavonoids (Mixed) | 50 mg |
| Alpha juice concentrate | 50 mg |
| Choline bitartrate | 30 mg |
| Inositol | 30 mg |
| Dong quai extract | 30 mg |
| Gingerroot extract | 30 mg |
| Licorice root extract | 30 mg |
| PABA | 30 mg |
| Chaste tree berry extract | 15 mg |
| Fennel seed extract | 15 mg |
| Carotenes | 5 mg |
| Boron | 3 mg |
| Silica | 1 mg |
| Vanadium | 50 mcg |

There are many good multiple vitamin/mineral formulas on the market today; however, there are also many inferior formulas. Be sure you choose a product that contains a good variety of essential nutrients at high enough levels. When choosing any nutritional supplements, utilize the advice in Chapter Three.

When deciding which nutritional supplements to take, an effective multiple vitamin/mineral formula is a great place to start. According to Dr. Judy Christianson, that's the first supplement she recommends for patients. "Most people are looking for more than just the prevention of vitamin deficiency diseases," explained Dr. Christianson. "A vitamin/mineral product that only contains 100 percent of the RDA may not be enough to support optimal health."

Dr. Michael Murray, recommends the following basic supplementation program:
- An effective multiple vitamin/mineral formula
- 1,000 to 3,000 mg of vitamin C daily
- 400 IU to 800 IU of vitamin E daily
- 1 to 2 tablespoons of Barlean's Flax Oil daily

His advice: "There are four cornerstones of good health," explains Dr. Murray, "a positive mental attitude, healthful diet, regular exercise, and supplementary measures."

Once again, there are two reasons why people search out natural health: prevention and treatment of a specific illness(es). Depending upon which category you are in, you will use therapeutic or mainte- nance dosages of nutritional supplements or specific nutrients. Maintenance dosages to help prevent illness and therapeutic dosages to help alleviate particular conditions.

Almost all disciplines within natural medicine have treatments that fall into one of these categories or a combination of both: therapeutic or maintenance. You can use natural medicine for either prevention or treatment of specific illnesses. Nutritional supplements operate on that same premise.

To get advice on how to use nutritional supplements for therapeutic purposes, you should visit a natural medicine provider. But remember, just as with any important decision in your life, take extra time to choose the right provider for your particular condition or purpose.

**Chapter summary**

Natural medicine provides a wide variety of treatments, prod- ucts, and services. You can use these to either prevent illness or treat disease. Nutritional supplements may be an area to explore considering the dietary habits of the general population.

We've discovered that unfortunately, RDAs are not accurate guide- lines when it comes to optimum nutrition. Because of a variety of factors, including stress, food processing, food additives, and other soci- etal trends, you may need to supplement your diet with nutritional products. Use care when choosing the right supplement and begin with a comprehensive multiple. From there, you will need to determine if you have specific symptoms or problems you need to address. Many nutritional formulas on the market today are designed to support different body functions.

Nutritional supplements are a great way to take control of your health. However, when there is a specific condition or set of symptoms present, consult a natural medicine healthcare professional. Chapter Five will tell you how to choose a natural medicine provider.

## My Supplement Plan

I am often asked what specific products I take to help boost my immune system and protect my body from cancer recurrence. Here is a list of products that I began taking as soon as I was diagnosed. This is a one year plan. After that, I will have my natural medicine physician contacts review what I should be taking as maintenance.

Keep in mind, we are all different. Although I feel this program works for me, it may not be the best for everyone. Remember, however, that whatever supplements you decide to take, your program will not be complete unless you incorporate a regular exercise program for your body and mind. Physical activity and attitude are so critical!

Vitamin C — 5 grams daily (Carlson Labs)
Beta carotene — 200,000 IU daily (Schiff)
Vitamin E — 800 IU daily (Carlson Labs)
EchinaFresh — 40 drops daily (Enzymatic Therapy)
OsteoPrime — 4 tablets daily (Enzymatic Therapy)
Pau D' Arco Tea — twice daily (Alta Health)
Essiac formula — as directed for three months only (Flora)
Doctor's Choice for Women — 3 tablets daily
(Enzymatic Therapy)
Fiber 6 — 3 tablets in a.m. before eating
(Simone Pharmaceuticals)
Mega-Zyme — 4 tablets twice daily on an empty stomach
(Enzymatic Therapy)
Ultra CoQ10 — 1/100 mg tablet daily (Twin Laboratories)

Remember, the dosages I am taking of many of these products is larger (therapeutic) doses because my body has experienced a crisis (cancer). If you are looking for more of a prevention program, the number of supplements you take and the dosages will not be this extensive. Visit your local health food store or a natural medicine healthcare provider for direction.

# CHAPTER FIVE

## How Do I Choose a Natural Medicine Provider?

Our present healthcare system has been overwhelmed by the practice of "disease management." As heart disease and cancer continue to eat away at the core of our quality of life escalating as our number one and two killers here in the United States, we continue to rely on reactive medicine rather than proactive preventive care.

The question remains: Are we tapping into all aspects of healthcare or are we so entrenched in conventional medical treatments that we are not seeing the complete picture? Where do "alternative" healthcare practices fit in the picture?

As consumers demand more from their healthcare system, they are finding that holistic healthcare is providing them with attractive alternatives they can use in conjunction with conventional medical care. Truly holistic healthcare efficiently utilizes the best of both worlds— conventional and alternative.

So far, we have learned that holistic healthcare is steeped in a strong tradition, based on scientific and anecdotal (testimonial) evidence, and is much safer than many of the conventional treatments available today. Holistic healthcare also emphasizes prevention rather than symptomatic relief. Holistic healthcare providers view the patient as a complicated puzzle consisting of many pieces rather than concentrating on just one piece as oftentimes happens with conventional medicine.

Holistic healthcare is about getting back to our roots—evaluating the patient as a complex individual by exploring all aspects of the human condition, rather than merely treating one or more symptoms. Getting back to basics and using the power within ourselves and the power of nature to help us stay healthy, gain better health, or rid our bodies of disease and illness—that's holistic healthcare.

Even our own government has admitted that nutritional supplements are important. Let's look at a specific government study proclaiming that nutrients will actually reverse the aging process and prevent disease as reported in the *Chicago Tribune* (3/26/93).

"Nutrition is today's new medicine," said Nancy Wellman of Florida International University. "There is increasing documentation that what you eat can make a big difference by speeding recovery times, shortening hospital stays and keeping people out of nursing homes." Wellman was one of the attendees at the United States Administration on Aging conference held in Chicago.

"What is exciting is that we are starting to get observations that say we should be able to delay or reverse many problems and symptoms associated with the aging process by increasing our intake of nutrients that are protective," said Dr. Irwin Rosenberg, director of the United States Department of Agriculture's Human Nutrition Research Center on Aging at Tufts University.

Ongoing government studies are confirming the possibility of preventing diseases that were once thought to be an inevitable part of growing old. Government nutritionists are also now recognizing the fact that nutritional supplementation may be necessary for those individuals who are not getting the appropriate nutrients from their diet.

According to Rosenberg, these are the newest government nutritional findings:
- vitamins E, B6, and zinc boost immunity in the elderly
- vitamins E, C, and beta carotene protect against heart disease, cancer, stroke, cataracts and other eye problems
- vitamins B6, B12, folate, calcium, potassium, and soluble fiber reduce the risk of heart disease
- vitamins B6, B12, and folate preserve mental alertness

Preventing disease through proper nutrition and possible supplementation can "help curb the nation's runaway healthcare costs," said Wellman. Many nutrition groups are already negotiating with insurance companies to have coverage extended to help the elderly who are malnourished gain proper nutritional status.

It is during times of stress that we often find out exactly how beneficial nutrition and nutritional supplementation is. Our country has been devastated by the onset of Acquired Immune Deficiency Syndrome (AIDS), a deadly virus that is growing in epidemic proportions. Even with this devastating disease, we are finding that specific nutrients can help prevent the disease from progressing.

Certain nutrients, taken in moderate to large doses, can slow the onset of full-blown AIDS in HIV-positive men. That's the conclusion of a study conducted by researchers at The Johns Hopkins Medical Institutions in Maryland.

The study, which was published in the December 1993 issue of the *American Journal of Epidemiology*, found that larger than usual amounts of vitamins A, C, B1, and niacin helped HIV-positive men remain free of AIDS for a significantly longer time than individuals taking smaller amounts of these nutrients. Of the 281 men participating in the study:

- Those who had a daily intake of more than 715 mg of vitamin C, 71.4 percent remained AIDS-free, while those who took less than 715 mg or less of vitamin C per day only 58.3 percent remained AIDS-free during the six-year study.
- Those who took more than 61 mg per day of niacin, 74.3 percent remained AIDS-free compared with 57.3 percent among those who took less than 61 mg daily of niacin.
- Those who had an intake of between 9,000 IU and 20,000 IU of vitamin A from food sources and supplements had a 45 percent decreased rate of AIDS progression; dosages above 20,000 IU seemed to actually diminish the effectiveness of this nutrient; well over 75 percent of the men in the study consumed over 180 percent of the Recommended Daily Allowance for vitamin A.
- Those who had a daily intake of over 4.9 mg of vitamin B1 also showed a significant slowed progression to AIDS.

The researchers concluded that vitamins A, C, B1, and niacin are important nutrients that can actually help slow the progression of developing full-blown AIDS for HIV-positive individuals.

"The effect we saw was quite substantial—a 40 percent to 48 percent decrease in new AIDS cases in this group that was sustained for more than six years," reported Alice M. Tang, M.S., the study's lead author. "If these results are confirmed by additional studies, we may have a useful intervention for HIV-positive patients."

The researchers concluded that nutrient intake must last for a minimum of two years to realize the benefit, and they recommend HIV-positive individuals start taking these nutrients as early as possible.

There is no longer a question of the beneficial effects specific nutrients and natural medicines can have on health and disease treatment. But what about holistic healthcare providers? How do they fit into this natural medicine menagerie of information? Who are these people? What can they do for us? And most of all, how can we pick the right provider?

Although there are never any easy answers when it comes to the complicated issue of health, there are some basics that will help you get started on the path to individual control.

It's about choice and it's about education—but most of all it's about our health. The single most important aspect of our lives, our health and the health of our family depends upon the decisions we make every day. Getting the proper information and assistance with those decisions is critical. Here's a look at the key holistic healthcare providers and the services they offer. You may want to recruit one or more of them in your search for health information.

**Acupuncture**

The mere thought of needles sends many people running in the opposite direction. However, acupuncture, which utilizes needles, does not hurt.

"With proper placement, you should feel a sensation, but no pain from the needle," explained Patricia Culliton, director of the Hennepin Faculty Associates Acupuncture and Alternative Medicine Clinic in Minnesota.

Acupuncture is designed to tap into the body's flow of energy. It originated in China and is based on the scientific belief that the body's energy flow determines proper function and may contribute either negatively or positively to your health. Literally hundreds of studies have confirmed that by inserting sterile, thin disposable needles into specific areas of the body, endorphins are released. Endorphins are powerful natural painkillers originating from the central nervous system.

Healthcare professionals utilizing acupuncture treatment may also recommend dietary modifications, nutritional supplements, specific exercises, and other lifestyle changes to enhance health or treat illness. Common conditions that respond very favorably to acupuncture treatments include back pain, chronic pain, and substance abuse. The World Health Organization has listed 41 different diseases that acupuncture treatments may help alleviate including PMS, gastrointestinal disorders, and respiratory illnesses to name a few.

The American Association of Acupuncture and Oriental Medicine (AAAOM) estimated that 12 million Americans received acupuncture treatment in 1994 alone. There are more than 50 acupuncture schools in the United States in addition to acupuncture courses offered at a few medical colleges. There are currently 7,000 licensed acupuncture practitioners in the United States, with more than 1,000 new practitioners being certified every year.

Presently, there are 30 states and the District of Columbia who license, certify, and register acupuncturists or officially recognize the practice of acupuncturists. Of these states, 22 register or certify acupuncturists for independent practice.

According to the AAAOM, private and public insurance coverage for acupuncture is available in many states. Medicaid covers this treatment for substance abuse in several states and Blue Cross/Blue Shield State Employee's Plans and Worker's Compensation also covers acupuncture treatments in several states. American Medical Security, a third-party insurance administrator located in Green Bay, WI has introduced a holistic healthcare plan that covers acupuncture treatments as well as most other natural treatments, products and services.

### Chiropractic care

No longer considered "alternative," chiropractic care has now become a key component within our healthcare system. In 1993, more than 45,000 licensed chiropractors were practicing in the United States. Currently, chiropractors see 12 percent to 15 percent of the United States population.

Chiropractic philosophy believes there is a strong correlation between body structure (primarily the spine) and body function (primarily the central nervous system). It is estimated that approximately one-half of the chiropractors in the United States utilize physical manipulation (also known as an adjustment), while the remainder utilize dietary modifications, nutritional supplements and other holistic treatment methods in addition to physical manipulation.

Many individuals use a chiropractor as their general physician. Chiropractors can and do treat a wide variety of illnesses; however, chiropractors do not prescribe medications or perform surgery. Chiropractic care is covered by most insurance companies.

## Clinical Nutrition Specialists

Nutrition plays a huge role in our health. What we eat and drink on a daily basis can make the difference between poor and peak performance. Healthcare professionals who specialize in nutritional counselling are called Certified Nutrition Specialists (C.N.S.).

Dr. Patrick Quillin holds a Ph.D., an R.D. (registered dietitian), and a C.N.S. Dr. Quillin, who is vice president of nutrition for the Cancer Treatment Centers of America and is the author of *Beating Cancer With Nutrition* (see appendix), says the C.N.S. is a relatively new program. The American College of Nutrition has a special division to certify C.N.S. candidates. Their criteria is strict and their procedure thorough.

"In general, graduates of these advanced degree programs (through The American College of Nutrition) have a higher level of competence and a broader scope of knowledge than do individuals who have not received formal training beyond the undergraduate level," according to The American College of Nutrition. Because of these high standards and the fact that this is a relatively new program, there are not many C.N.S. professionals available. Don't be confused by people who have C.N. after their names or simply call themselves nutritionists. Dr. Quillin explains that these individuals are not certified by The American College of Nutrition, which is the only organization that specializes in strictly monitored certification.

The C.N.S. professional is able to diagnose, assess, and treat a wide variety of conditions using nutrition and nutritional status as a foundation. "...the use of individual nutrients in therapeutic amounts (large) increasingly is becoming incorporated into mainstream medical treatment and health maintenance," concluded The American College of Nutrition. "These trends in modern scientific disease prevention and treatment have increased the demand for innovative, responsible, and creative professional nutritionists."

As with any other natural medicine provider, when choosing a nutritionist, be sure to find out exactly how they have been trained. Often, you will find a medical doctor (M.D.) or a doctor of osteopathic medicine (D.O.) who specializes in the practice of nutritional therapy. These healthcare professionals have chosen the science of nutrition as their specialty and should be able to provide you with effective service.

### Homeopathy

Homeopathic medicine has a long-standing history within the United States. By the close of the 19th century, there were 22 homeopathic medical schools, more than 100 homeopathic hospitals, and approximately 15 percent of the physician population was practicing homeopathy.

"The practice of homeopathy (along with other types of alternative medicine) declined dramatically in the United States following the publication of the *Flexner Report* in 1910, which established guidelines for the funding of medical schools," according to *Alternative Medicine: Expanding Medical Horizons*, a report prepared for the National Institutes of Health. The newly established guidelines favored the American Medical Association's standards and virtually crippled competing schools of medicine, including homeopathic colleges.

Within the past decade there has been an escalated interest in homeopathy because of the results achieved and the low toxicity. Homeopathic science contends that the body's immune system can fight illness if given the chance. It is a highly individualized form of medicine that works with each person's unique chemistry.

In homeopathic treatment, the patient is given a formula with one or more highly diluted natural ingredient(s) that would cause the same symptoms of the condition if given in large dosages. It can be compared to a vaccine in that the formula stimulates the body's immune system to fight off the illness. Homeopathy can be used for acute or chronic illnesses as well as for prevention and health promotion purposes. Many homeopathic formulations, which are made from naturally occurring plant, animal, or mineral substances, are over-the-counter approved in the United States.

Because the active component of the homeopathic formula is so diluted (oftentimes, not even detectable through current scientific methods), some conventional medical practitioners reject homeopathy. Homeopathy, however, not only has a long history of use, it is also supported by many clinical studies. In 1992, the *British Medical Journal* conducted an evaluation of 22 well-designed scientific studies and found that 15 of the 22 showed positive results, indicating that homeopathy provides therapeutic benefits to those who use the formulations.

"Homeopathic remedies are recognized and regulated by the Food and Drug Administration and are manufactured by established pharmaceutical companies under strict guidelines established by the Homeopathic Pharmacopoeia of the United States," according to *Alternative Medicine: Expanding Medical Horizons.* "Recent surveys in the United States found that most homeopathic patients seek care for chronic illnesses and that homeopathic physicians spend twice as much time with their patients, order half as many laboratory tests and procedures, and prescribe fewer drugs."

Although homeopathy remains somewhat controversial within the conventional medical establishment, positive clinical studies have been published in such highly regarded medical journals as the *Lancet*, the *British Medical Journal*, and the *American Academy of Pediatrics*. Because the homeopathic concept of "less is more" contradicts with our conventional medical establishment, there will no doubt continue to be controversy surrounding homeopathy; however, we should take the advice from one *Lancet* article headline which read—*Homeopathy: Keeping an open mind.*

Approximately 3,000 physicians and other healthcare practitioners presently use homeopathy. In 1990, it was estimated that about one percent of the United States population, 2.5 million people, utilized the services of a homeopathic doctor. Homeopathic licensing varies from state-to-state. Homeopathic healthcare providers typically couple this service with other degrees including medical, osteopathic, and naturopathic.

## Naturopathic medicine

"Naturopathic medicine is a distinct primary healthcare profession emphasizing prevention, treatment and optimal health through the use of therapeutic methods and substances which encourage the person's inherent self-healing process," according to the American Association of Naturopathic Physicians (AANP).

Naturopathic physicians use nutritional and herbal medicines, lifestyle counselling, homeopathy, acupuncture, minor surgery and homeopathy to treat their patients for a wide variety of conditions. Doctors of Naturopathic Medicine (N.D.s) use all methods of clinical and laboratory diagnostic testing just as conventional doctors do.

"Naturopathic physicians are more concerned with finding the underlying cause of a condition and applying treatments that work in alliance with the natural healing mechanisms of the body rather than against them," according to the AANP. "Naturopathic treatments result less frequently in adverse side effects, or in the chronic conditions that inevitably arise when the cause of the disease is left untreated."

Naturopathic physicians are trained to make the appropriate referrals just as conventional medical doctors. Naturopathic medicine is typically used in nonemergency situations. The biggest difference between naturopathic physicians and conventional medical doctors is their philosophy. The principles of naturopathic medicine include:

- *The healing power of nature.* According to the AANP, naturopathic physicians work to restore and support the patient's inherent healing abilities.
- *First do no harm.* N.D.s prefer to utilize noninvasive treatments which tend to minimize the risks of harmful side effects.
- *Find the cause.* Finding the underlying cause of a condition is a key goal of the naturopathic physician.
- *Treat the whole person.* Health or disease comes from a complex interaction of physical, emotional, dietary, genetic, environmental, lifestyle, and other factors.
- *Preventive medicine.* The naturopathic goal is to prevent minor illnesses from developing into more serious or chronic, degenerative diseases.

Naturopathic medicine has been a recognized American medical profession since 1902. Presently, there are ten states that license naturopathic physicians. There are two accredited colleges of Naturopathic Medicine in the United States: Bastyr University in Seattle, WA, and National College in Portland, OR. Southwest College of Naturopathic Medicine and Health Sciences in Scottsdale, AZ, is a candidate for accreditation. These naturopathic medicine colleges are four-year postgraduate schools with admissions requirements comparable to those of conventional medical schools. The N.D. degree requires four years of graduate level study in the medical sciences.

It is important to emphasize that naturopathic physicians who hold degrees from other organizations do not have the same professional training as naturopathic doctors who graduate from one of the accredited colleges.

"Unfortunately, some people obtain questionable N.D. degrees from brief correspondence courses, short seminars, or from schools that give credit for live experience but which do not require clinical training," warns the AANP. "Such degrees are usually not recognized by state degree-authorizing bodies."

To help protect consumers, the AANP supports legislation to license N.D.s in all states in order to distinguish properly trained physicians from less qualified individuals. AANP membership is limited to individuals who are eligible for licensing in states which issue licenses.

Naturopathic medicine is covered by many insurance carriers including the new American Medical Security HealthCareChoice$ plan. According to the AANP, Connecticut and Alaska have mandated insurance reimbursement for medically necessary and appropriate naturopathic medical services.

## Osteopathic medicine

A D.O. is a doctor of osteopathic medicine. Osteopathic physicians are qualified to provide complete healthcare to the patient. No longer considered "alternative," osteopathic medicine incorporates virtually all branches of medical science. Osteopathic medicine combines both conventional and holistic philosophies in an effort to provide quality healthcare.

"Osteopathic medicine is a system of medical care with a philosophy that combines the needs of the patient with the current practice of medicine, surgery and obstetrics with an emphasis on the inter-relationship of structure and function and with an appreciation of the body's ability to heal itself," states the American Osteopathic Association (AOA).

Presently, there are 16 AOA-accredited colleges throughout the United States. Typically, students who enroll in one of the accredited colleges hold a bachelor's degree. To gain a doctorate in osteopathic medicine, four years of study in an osteopathic medical school is required.

Here are some more facts about osteopathic medicine as provided by the AOA:

- By the year 2000, it is expected that 45,000 osteopathic physicians will be in practice in the United States.
- Over half of all D.O.s practice in the primary care areas of general practice, internal medicine, obstetrics/gynecology and pediatrics.
- D.O.s represent 5.5 percent of the total United States physician population and 10 percent of all United States military physicians.
- Each year, ten million patient visits are made to D.O.s.

"You are more than just the sum of your body. That's why doctors of osteopathic medicine practice a whole person approach to medicine," concluded the AOA. "Instead of just treating specific symptoms, osteopathic physicians concentrate on treating you as a whole."

D.O.s are licensed to perform surgery and prescribe medication in all 50 states. The AOA represents the more than 36,000 D.O.s across the United States. It is estimated that 69 percent of the nation's D.O.s are members of the AOA.

### Buyer beware...

When we buy a car or a piece of real estate, we ask a lot of questions, right? After all, we don't want to waste our good, hard-earned money on a bad investment. The only difference between your health and buying a car or a home is that your health is so much more important. That means you should be even more cautious and ask even more questions.

Choosing a healthcare provider is an important decision—holistic providers are no exception. Here are some tips you can use to pick the provider that's best for you.

**1. You're in charge.** Recognize that you are the boss and you need to feel comfortable. You are the healthcare customer and you can refuse service, change providers, and question treatments.

**2. Determine what you need.** You need to decide what type of provider you are looking for: general practitioner; Ob/Gyn; allergist; etc. You will have a better idea after you write down your goals and complete the head-to-toe evaluation featured in Chapter Three.

**3. Make a connection.** You need to be able to communicate comfortably with your provider. Make sure you pick a provider that will listen to your needs and evaluate you as a person, not just a symptom. Personality is important. If you don't connect with the first doctor you've chosen, don't feel bad—just pick another one. Never settle for someone you can't "connect" with and who is not sensitive to your needs.

**4. Ask questions.** Don't be afraid to ask about your doctor's professional credentials. Where did they get their degree? Do they belong to any professional organizations? Are they certified with the state? Trust your intuition. If anything seems amiss, pick another provider. Be sure that the doctor you choose is willing and able to work with other physicians if necessary. A physician should not be intimidated by second opinions or reluctant to make referrals to specialists. When I was first diagnosed with cancer, I told my oncologist (a doctor that was just "assigned" to me; I didn't choose him) that I was going to get a second opinion from the University of Wisconsin-Madison hospital and that I was going to fax my reports to my natural medicine doctors. His response was the best: "Great! I think the more input we get about your case, the better off we will be." He encouraged my involvement. Needless to say, I was glad he was assigned to my case.

**5. Above all, educate yourself.** Before you even pick a provider, learn more about their specialty. Learn more about your own condition. Learn more about your body and the signals it sends you. You are the commander. To lead yourself on your health journey, you need to learn as much as you can about your journey. The success of holistic healthcare depends largely on you and how informed you are. Even after selecting a provider, continue your educational process. You'll probably find the learning an enjoyable and empowering process.

Be sure to pick a provider that has your best interest in mind at all times. Let your intuition be your best friend. If you have a bad feeling about any part of your healthcare, bring it up to your physician and if it does not get resolved the way you want, choose a different healthcare provider.

In order to experience success with a holistic healthcare provider, you will need to get to know your provider as they get to know you. Make your choice wisely. This is an important decision, so don't take it lightly and don't take anything for granted. Just because a doctor has a degree does not make him/her a good doctor. Consider this: The People's Medical Society, a national medical consumer group, has estimated that at least 80,000 people die each year from medical negligence. Another 300,000 receive serious injuries that often lead to permanent disability. Medication errors are also far too commonplace. At Mass General Hospital in New York each year, there are 500 preventable medication errors, which can cause serious harm or even death—and that's just *one* hospital. There is no question that if you aren't already sick, choosing the wrong doctor could really make you sick.

Information is power. Gather as much information before choosing a specific provider or treatment. Check with your insurance carrier if you need to find out if a treatment or service is covered.

### More choices

There have been literally hundreds of chapters written on holistic healthcare treatments and providers. Although not everything written has been positive, the proper information does exist. It's up to you to do the research.

Recognize that you have more choices than you may realize. Take the time to do the "legwork." When you invest the time, you are making the most important investment of your life—your health just may depend upon it.

One of the biggest myths about holistic healthcare is that it is "on the fringe." That it's not sophisticated or scientific. The fact remains, however, that holistic healthcare philosophies and treatment practices have been embraced for centuries as a key mode of healthcare delivery.

"Worldwide, only an estimated 10 percent to 30 percent of human healthcare is delivered by conventional, biomedically oriented practitioners," according to the report to the National Institutes of Health (NIH), *Alternative Medicine: Expanding Medical Horizons.* "The remaining 70 percent to 90 percent ranges from self-care according to folk principles to care given in an organized healthcare system based on an alternative tradition or practice."

The *Alternative Medicine* report to the NIH concluded that the alternative therapies and practices they reviewed "represent a great and largely untapped resource for improving the nation's health."

Although far from perfect, holistic healthcare providers are offering more options to individuals looking for effective, less toxic, more personal alternatives. To our ailing healthcare system, holistic health-care providers offer treatments that are more economical. Most important, to the consumer willing to do the research and take the time to determine what's best for them, holistic healthcare offers more choices.

## Chapter summary

We've learned about some of the key natural medicine practitioners and the services they offer. There are natural medicine providers who offer services for virtually all conditions, except emergency/crisis care (i.e. bleeding, loss of consciousness, paralysis, etc.).

Remember that you are in charge of the relationship. As the healthcare customer, you can change doctors at any time. Choosing your doctor is one of the most important decisions you will make—be sure you are comfortable with your choice.

Ask lots of questions not only of the doctor, but also other people. Ask friends if they've seen the doctor and what they've heard about the doctor. You may even want to call your insurance company to get their input.

Now, it's time to take all the information you've learned and move on to bigger and better things.

# CHAPTER SIX

## What's The Next Step?

S o far, we've learned a lot of positive facts about natural medicine; however, there is something else you also need to know: People usually don't find out about all of the alternatives available until the crisis is nearly out of control. In many cases, natural medicine is chosen as a last resort instead of a weapon of first choice.

Fortunately, this trend is changing. Many healthcare professionals, patients, and health writers (including myself) feel the tide is turning toward more effective usage of and information about natural medicine. Natural medicine is being viewed as a valuable component of our healthcare system. Consumers are taking control just as you have done by reading this book. We are all hungry for more information about how we can stay healthy or rid our bodies of illness by using the least toxic, most effective, economical methods. Natural medicine provides us with viable alternatives.

### Education is everything

In order for your healthcare to be truly effective, you need to get involved. And that means educate yourself on all forms of healthcare— natural and conventional. No, you don't have to have a medical degree to become educated on health, but you do need to have these characteristics:

- Be inquisitive and ask lots of questions.
- Be assertive and don't be intimidated.

• Communicate your needs clearly and frankly.

And remember, education is an ongoing process. I have been fortunate to attend a wide variety of natural medicine conferences, seminars, and trade shows over the years. Each time I go to an event, I always manage to learn something new.

Always keep yourself open to new learning opportunities. You'll be surprised just how much valuable health information is available.

David Ellig has written a great book on patient education (mostly regarding conventional healthcare; however, much of his advice applies to natural medicine as well), *Never Get Naked On Your First Visit* (see appendix). Ellig explains that the following results have been proven when a patient is more educated and receives more information:

• Nearly 26 percent fewer hysterectomies.
• 33 percent fewer hospital admittances for asthmatics.
• Patients with high blood pressure and diabetes had lower, more favorable readings.
• 60 percent fewer prostate surgeries.
• A 15 percent reduction in drug costs.

Here is Ellig's "healthcare consumer statement of beliefs:"

1) We recognize that we are extremely vulnerable when we require medical services and expect that our healthcare givers will treat us in a caring, open and honest manner.
2) We recognize that we hire doctors, hospitals and labs to provide services for our most important possessions—our lives and those of our family and friends.
3) We pay substantial fees for these services.
4) We have a right to expect services and skill levels to be commensurate with the price of services.
5) We have the right to determine the quality of the provider of our services.
6) We recognize that medical services cannot be provided without our permission and we will not be asked to give approval until we fully understand the qualifications of the provider, and the services to be provided, and our expectations agree with the provider's expectations.
7) We recognize that only those services we agree to may be provided.
8) We recognize that by accepting this statement of beliefs we

may discover some facts that we don't want to know, but would rather discover those facts before treatment rather than after treatment.

"Finally, we recognize that our interest in our medical treatment is greater than that of the healthcare giver; it is our life and lifestyle at risk, it is their vocation," concluded Ellig. "We expect the healthcare giver to put our interest before their own."

Of course, these beliefs do not come without responsibility from you, the patient (i.e. healthcare consumer). I propose that you make the following promises to yourself and your healthcare provider(s):

1) Educate yourself about your health by doing a thorough head-to-toe evaluation and health history so you recognize important signals about your present health status before visiting a healthcare provider or purchasing natural medicine products and services. It will also be a great idea to start (or add to your present) health library; it's good to have the proper information right at your fingertips. And never forget about your local library (or your local hospital's library), or now, the internet. A wealth of information exists out there; you just need to tap into it!

2) Put your health at the top of your priority list and never lose sight of the importance of your health. By doing so, you will be sending a strong message to those who support you in that goal—family, friends, and providers. I suggest putting your health goals in writing, including specifics about diet and exercise. Review your goals daily if possible and share them with the people you love.

3) Trust your intuition and never stop learning about your health and the health of those you love.

4) If your healthcare provider becomes intimidated by your involvement in your healthcare, switch providers immediately. You are the employer and you need to be in control.

Being in control is so important when it comes to your health. When my mom was diagnosed with terminal cancer, there was nothing anyone could do. Her pancreatic cancer was so advanced that the doctors gave her only three months to live. We contacted our local Hospice to help us monitor her pain medication and keep her as comfortable as possible. She needed around the clock care. My sister and I took turns staying with her. One of the feelings I had during this traumatic time was the feeling of helplessness. Her cancer was so out of control that it controlled us. We were prisoners to this disease. I never want to experience that loss of control or helplessness again.

Today, I have learned that the way we view life and our attitude affect how fulfilling our lives will be. It was quite clear that my mom was ready to die, so she gave up her fight and let the rest in God's hand.

There is no doubt that the state of your mind will have an influence on your health outcome. For my mom, she wanted to die quickly once she discovered she could not have the quality of life she had enjoyed. She began to pray that God would take her—and he did, on January 6, just three weeks after her diagnosis.

Your psychological status before, during and after illness should not be ignored. There was an interesting study done on women who had cancer to explore the effects psychological intervention would have on their survival outcome. The study, conducted by English researcher Steve Greer, found that the way the woman chooses to respond to her condition (in the case of this study, it was breast cancer) affects her survival outcome more than any other single factor, including the initial stage of her cancer.

Greer's study, which lasted 15 years, found that patients with a fighting attitude had the best chance of survival. Those in denial also did well. Indifferent acceptance (an I-don't-care attitude) lowered the chance of survival. And a helpless/hopeless attitude had the worst chance for survival. This study illustrates the importance of being in control of your health, rather than letting an illness control you.

Even more important, Greer's follow-up work has shown that cancer patients improve with psychological counselling. "In other words, you aren't stuck with a poor attitude just because it's habitual. The improvement included more fighting spirit, the very attitude associated with the longest survival," writes Steve Austin, N.D. in his book *Breast Cancer: What You Should Know (But May Not Be Told) About Prevention, Diagnosis, and Treatment* (see appendix). He and his wife Cathy Hitchcock, who is a breast cancer survivor, did an outstanding job on this book. I feel it is the best book written on breast cancer because it merges the emotional with the conventional, and the natural. It's an excellent book. Dr. Judy Christianson gave that book to my sister after her diagnosis and what a great gift it was! I liked the book so much that I called Steve and Cathy and asked them if IMPAKT could distribute it. Fortunately, they said yes.

Being in control does not mean that you are pushy or obnoxious. It means that you are confident and eager for information. Always try to keep your composure. Remember, no question is a bad question. If you are too shy or embarrassed to ask a question, have a friend or family member do it for you. The objective is to always receive an answer that you can understand. If you don't understand the response, say so. Embarrassment won't kill you, but misinformation and lack of education could!

Being a wise healthcare consumer means weighing the pros and cons and thinking through your decisions. For example, going to the emergency room in the middle of the night for a stuffy head is probably not a good idea. Take some extra vitamin C, maybe a homeopathic cold formula, and call your doctor in the morning if necessary. Being a wise healthcare consumer means evaluating the emotional as well as financial ramifications of your decisions.

As our country's healthcare tab escalates to one trillion dollars, we all need to be conscious of how our healthcare choices affect the entire system. Just by doing the proper research prior to receiving medical treatment can have huge financial implications. Let me give you an example. If you are diagnosed with a peptic ulcer and given a prescription for Tagamet or Zantac, recognize that you do not have to take the prescription. After visiting a natural medicine practitioner, you would be given the following treatment plan for your peptic ulcer:
- a diet recommendation of more fiber
- you would be told to stop smoking, if you do
- you would be given stress reduction techniques
- you would be told to get more of certain nutrients (vitamins A, C, and E, and zinc)
- you would be given DGL (which has been shown to be more effective and much safer than Tagamet, Zantac or antacids)

Tagamet and Zantac typically cost over $100 a month, while DGL is available for about $15 a month. Tagamet and Zantac have a high relapse rate because it merely works to correct symptoms, while DGL helps repair the damaged stomach lining. As you can see, the decision to go the natural route has not only saved money, it will be better for your health in the long run.

With managed care and insurance prices continuing to escalate, the days of "Oh, my insurance will pay for it" are over. I know first hand, how financially challenging it can be to have a serious illness. That's why it's more important than ever to exercise some common sense when it comes to the decisions you make regarding your health.

## Our healthcare crisis

Our present medical system is one of the finest, most technologically advanced healthcare programs in the world. And yet, according to a disturbing report by the World Health Organization, in the early 1990s the United States ranked 24th in national healthcare and 19th in infant survival rate. Babies in 18 other countries survive longer than the infants born in the United States.

The treatment of chronic, degenerative diseases such as heart disease, cancer, and arthritis, account for 85 percent of the national healthcare bill. Fairly new illnesses such as environmental illness, chronic fatigue, and AIDS are plaguing this country. Although our current conventional medical system is great at managing medical emergencies, certain bacterial infections, trauma care, and many complex surgical techniques, it fails miserably in the areas of preventing diseases and managing chronic illnesses.

"We wait for it (illness) to develop and then spend huge sums on heroic measures, even then ignoring the underlying lifestyle-related causes," concluded the American Association of Naturopathic Physicians. "This is the equivalent of waiting for a leaky roof to destroy the infrastructure of a house and then repairing the damage without fixing the leak. This is naturally expensive and ineffective."

Ironically, we often use more common sense and take more control over issues involving our car or our house than our irreplaceable bodies. We need to remember our priorities and give our health the time and attention it deserves.

I believe one of the reasons we have such an expensive healthcare system is because we are not utilizing all of the choices that are available. Often we are not looking at the whole picture. In order for truly effective healthcare to take place, we need to merge the conventional with the natural. We need to emphasize lifestyle factors and concentrate on preventing illness. If we begin to practice preventive medicine rather than reactive crisis management, we just may put a dent in the trillion dollar healthcare tab that continues to climb.

Our present healthcare crisis has caused a shift—a new way of thinking. We're adopting a more open-minded, all-inclusive, comprehensive, holistic way of thinking. And fortunately, you are at the helm steering this message home. You will not stand for inadequate care, but you will also do your part to take care of your health and the health of your family as much as humanly possible. You will contribute to our ailing healthcare system in a positive, constructive manner. And that just may include trying many natural medicine concepts, treatments, products, or services.

While there has been negative publicity causing more confusion about natural medicine, the positive media attention cannot be overlooked. Countless mainstream magazines, newspapers, television shows, and radio programs have been eager to confirm what "alternative" physicians have known for centuries: Nature's medicine cabinet can be very powerful.

In late 1992, *The New York Times* magazine promoted alternative medicine in their two-part series dealing with everything from acupuncture to biofeedback, homeopathy to naturopathy.

"The importance of this article (in *The New York Times*) is that it is one of a number of pieces to occur in mainstream publications with a large circulation and high credibility that focuses on the fact that herbs and other alternative modalities are gaining increasing mainstream acceptance, not only by consumers who appear to be fueling the interest in natural healthcare, but also among conventional physicians and other health professionals," said Mark Blumenthal, executive director of the American Botanical Council, a nonprofit herbal research organization. Blumenthal cites the Dan Rather CBS evening news week-long series regarding "alternative medicine" as still another example of positive media attention.

Much of the media attention of late has focused on the FDA's wish to reduce consumer access to information and natural products themselves. Fear of losing the right to choose and use many nutritional supplements has caused much political debate. Regarding herbal medicines, it was reported in the *Chicago Sun Times* that Purdue University Professor Varro E. Tyler would like to see "the FDA develop a sensible regulatory process that at the same time would not deny consumers access to these products." The Dietary Supplement Bill, passed in

Congress in May 1994, is supposed to be that "sensible" piece of legislation regarding the regulation of nutritional supplements.

The huge consumer grassroots effort to ensure passage of The Dietary Supplement Bill has fueled much of the renewed interest and in natural medicine causing increased media attention.

"Consumers need protection from drugs and doctors, not supplements and alternative care," according to an article promoting natural medicine in *The Nation*, a leading magazine of political and social commentary.

Still another article appearing in *Natural Health* magazine, poses the commonly asked question, "Why are doctors blind to the well-documented research about vitamins?"

In *Utne Reader* magazine, homeopathic educator and author Dana Ullman concludes, "When American doctors start saying that they've supported alternative medicine all along, they'll be faking it—but we'll all be better off."

It seems as though the tide is turning. More and more consumers, research scientists, medical doctors, and other health professionals are starting to recognize the truly therapeutic value of the many health alternatives that are available.

Early in 1994, the editors of the University of California, Berkley *Wellness Letter* also jumped on the vitamin bandwagon. According to an article in the January 1994 issue, although the editorial board "has been reluctant to recommend supplementary vitamins on a broad scale," they have now changed that position.

"The accumulation of research in recent years has caused us to change our minds—at least where four vitamins are concerned," according to the editors of the *Wellness Letter*. The vitamins they are now promoting are the antioxidant vitamins E and C, beta carotene, and the B vitamin, folic acid (also known as folacin). The editors explained, "...even if you do eat a very healthy diet—and most Americans do not—it's unlikely you will get the high levels of folacin and the antioxidant vitamins many authorities think you need."

The *Wellness Letter* reported that a high intake of these antioxidant vitamins "seems to be protective against many kinds of cancer. The role these substances play in disease prevention is no longer a matter of dispute."

"For all that science can disclose, the body retains its mysteries," wrote Adriane Fugh-Berman, M.D. in *The Nation*. "Perhaps one day we will be privileged to have a medical system that encourages humility among doctors, and uses the most benign therapy that is effective for each medical condition. That would truly be a revolution in healthcare."

There is no question that natural medicine options are becoming more respected and more utilized. An example of this is that many of the services, treatments and products discussed in this book are now covered by some insurance companies. I have been fortunate to consult with American Medical Security, a third-party insurance administrator located in Green Bay, WI, on their holistic health insurance product. The product, called HealthCareChoice$, is one of the first truly comprehensive plans to cover alternative healthcare. When I first heard about the plan, I was afraid American Medical Security was going to be like the many other insurance firms that have tried to cover natural medicine—they "cherry pick" treatments and services only choosing those that provide benefit to the insurance company rather than the insured. American Medical Security chose not to just "dabble" in this area; instead they jumped in with both feet. I compliment American Medical Security on this innovative new concept. For more information on HealthCareChoice$, refer to the appendix of this book.

Natural medicine surely does not provide us with all of the answers. But, what if it provides us with some of the answers? Can we afford to overlook the possible benefits in the face of such a national crisis? It's about options and about choice. The more weapons we have in our fight to gain better health and treat disease, the better off we will be.

It is clear that holistic healthcare isn't just for a select group of visionaries anymore. There are colleges and organizations dedicated to studying it and there are qualified healthcare professionals willing to practice it. Most importantly, there are Americans who are demanding it.

When discussing natural medicine, this quote by Thomas Edison is often used: "The doctor of the future will give no medicine, but will interest his patients in the care of the human frame, in diet, and in the cause and prevention of disease." The reason this quote is so frequently used is because 1) Thomas Edison is, of course, highly respected and

2) he made this successful prediction a very long time ago. Thomas Edison is clearly describing natural medicine.

However, in order for any healthcare concept to be successful, you need to be the primary player. Take part in your healthcare because if you don't get involved, you just may suffer the consequences.

Truly comprehensive healthcare involves both the conventional and natural. Although some services may not interest you, keep an open mind and do your homework. You can pick and choose based upon the knowledge you gain as an educated healthcare consumer.

## An exciting journey

Now that you have the basics of natural medicine, you are on your way to a world filled with fascinating facts, interesting testimonials and viable alternatives. Don't let it overwhelm you. Embrace the information and enjoy the ride. Your journey will introduce you to many interesting people and new ideas. I cherish the friendships I have made during my exploration of natural medicine. My interviews and meetings with people like Dr. Linus Pauling, Naomi Judd, Mark Victor Hansen (author of *Chicken Soup for the Soul*), and others have been inspirational. Most of all, I have enjoyed talking to our readers, people like you who have experienced the frustration, fear, and determination that can come with healthcare.

But remember: Just as with any trip, chart your course wisely. Be an active healthcare consumer, not a passive patient who blindly listens to anything or anyone. Be eager, not naive.

Your next step is to take on more advanced reading material. Go over the terms in the glossary section of this book and then choose a book(s) that pique your interest. Take advantage of the information provided in the appendix of this book—*help yourself* to the information available to you.

Here are two books that I recommend you start with. No home should be without either:

1. *Alternative Medicine: The Definitive Guide* compiled by the Burton Goldberg Group. I met Burton Goldberg and was impressed by his commitment to this cause. He invested two million dollars of his own money to get the book to the marketplace. The contributor's list reads like the "who's who" of natural medicine. This book features advice from 350 leading natural medicine healthcare providers on a

wide variety of conditions. It's a great reference book (all 1,068 pages of it).

2. *Natural Alternatives to Over-the-Counter and Prescription Drugs* by Michael T. Murray, N.D. is truly a one-of-a-kind work. Dr. Murray provides readers with the information they are looking for: How to avoid drug therapy or replace drug therapy with safer, natural alternatives. This reference book includes alternatives to common drugs such as Tagamet, Prednisone, Zantac, Cardisem, and 208 other prescription drugs, as well as natural alternatives to over-the-counter drugs used to treat acne, high cholesterol, insomnia, arthritis, headache, and many other common health conditions. Dr. Murray is one of the finest natural medicine researchers of our time. With this book, he has proven that he is a premier natural medicine author.

**Chapter summary**

If your healthcare program is going to work, you need to take charge. Never stop learning and never accept complacency from your healthcare providers. We are in the midst of a very serious healthcare crisis. Together we can make a difference and arm ourselves against disease. If each one of us thoroughly evaluates our healthcare decisions, the ripple effect will be more powerful than any managed care concept presented.

It's time to help yourself to some good, old-fashioned healthy living. *Help yourself* to the information that's available to you. And most of all, *help yourself* to the world of natural medicine—providing you with effective, safe healthcare choices.

You've taken your important first steps, but remember you need to walk before you can run. Be cautious on your journey. Each step you take will provide you with a great deal of information. Sift through the information, only keeping what will help you accomplish your health goals.

Congratulations and welcome to the world of natural medicine. Good luck in your search for good health. The more you learn, the more you can *help yourself* and the people you love.

# FINAL THOUGHTS

When we were thinking of a title for this book, everyone agreed that *Help Yourself* was the most appropriate. That's what truly effective healthcare is all about: Helping ourselves to effective treatments, services, products, and information. The title is even more fitting because the natural medicine philosophy has been built on what I call "medical hospitality." Natural medicine practitioners invite you into their clinics and spend quality time with you to learn more about your needs and health goals. There is something appealing about healthcare with a smile and receiving information from people who truly care about you.

This "medical hospitality" is beginning to seep into all aspects of our healthcare system because we as consumers are demanding it. Our conventional establishment is learning that there is more to healthcare than reacting once disease has struck. We are all realizing that we play a vital role in our health and the health of those we love.

Healthcare is not a spectator sport. This old saying rings true: You gotta play the game if you're going to win. To be in the healthcare game, you need to be an active participant knowing what you need in order to win. It just may be time for you to put natural medicine on your team.

Natural medicine has a respected history of use and most treatments, services, and products have been validated by hard science. In addition, literally millions of people all over the world have benefitted from natural medicine. I have been fortunate to have the opportunity to talk with people every week who have experienced the power of natural medicine.

I have also listened to their stories of desperation. The story of the woman whose 26-year-old pregnant daughter found out she had cancer. Another mother who lost her only daughter to cancer. The son who cares for his mother with Alzheimer's. A father whose son had bone cancer and was searching for something to help his child. The mother who watches her child with AIDS waste away. The man who nearly died from a heart attack. The young man with lung cancer who was given just months to live, but beat his cancer and remains healthy today.

So many people wrote to me after my mom died, just to let me know that they too had lost their mom at a very young age. They knew my pain first-hand. The pain of disease and illness cannot be described.

Just as we need to educate ourselves on health, so too, we need to learn about death and dying. It's a topic not often discussed (especially in a book about health), but it's an issue we all must face. There is really no getting around it. A good friend of mine explains it this way: We all need to answer for the lives we've led when the final invoice comes due.

I don't look at my mom's death as our failure to save her. Although I miss her desperately and wish she were "physically" here with us, she taught me that it's all part of the package. With life comes death. While she was dying, she taught me more about life than I could have ever learned from a textbook or a seminar. She taught me to live my life with passion and commitment. She told me never to take more than I can give. "Work hard and play hard," that's the way she wanted me to live my life. But, she also taught me to value my health more than anything else.

When my sister was diagnosed with breast cancer, it was so traumatic for my mom. She always lived her life for her six children and 11 grandchildren. She was such a devoted mother and grandmother. Her final messages to us were to take care of each other and take care of our health.

I have discovered that good health doesn't just mean fewer medical bills or "just" making it through the day. Good health means vitality. It helps you accomplish your dreams and live life to the fullest.

I have made the commitment to do everything in my power to protect my health and help create optimum health. For me, that includes utilizing natural medicine.

My goal is that you can see the value in exploring all of your options regarding your healthcare. Recognize that you have many choices. You will be able to determine which choice is the most valid and appropriate for you based on your needs and health goals. It all comes down to results and not settling for complacency.

Because my mom was such a big part of this book (although it occurred after her death), I would like to close with the advice she often gave me. Apply it to your health and to your life. Use what you can, disregard the rest:

- Treat people with respect and they will treat you with respect.
- You can accomplish anything you put your mind to.
- Always believe in yourself and the power that lies within you.

When my mom walked into a room, it lit up with her smile and her sparkling blue eyes. Her energy and enthusiasm were contagious. She made people feel good and always left them a little happier than they were before.

This is the legacy that she leaves behind. Thank you for letting her touch your life.

Know what's important in life: Family, friends, faith, and most of all, health! Do all you can to protect each of these and you will find true happiness.

# APPENDIX

## Natural Medicine References

## Magazines/newsletters

*Health Counselor*
P.O. Box 12496
Green Bay, WI 54307-2496
1-800-477-2995
$18/year (six issues per year)
A consumer magazine detailing advances in natural health and nutrition.

*Health Security*
P.O. Box 12496
Green Bay, WI 54307-2496
1-800-477-2995
$12/year (six issues per year)
The only corporate wellness magazine that features a section on natural medicine.

*The American Journal of Natural Medicine*
P.O. Box 12496
Green Bay, WI 54307-2496
1-800-477-2995
$59/year (ten issues per year)
The physician's guide to clinical research.

*Nutrition News* by Siri Khalsa
4108 Watkins Dr.
Riverside, CA 92507
(909) 784-7500
$18/year (twelve issues per year)
A monthly four-page newsletter for consumers that discusses natural medicine alternatives for specific conditions.

*Health & Healing Newsletter* by Dr. Julian Whitaker
Phillips Publishing
1-800-777-5005
$39.95/year (twelve issues per year)

*Alternative Medicine Digest* by the Burton Goldberg Group
$18/year (six issues per year)
1-800-720-6363

*The Journal of Orthomolecular Medicine*
16 Florence Ave.
Toronto, Ontario, Canada M2N 1E9
(416) 733-2117 FAX (416) 733-2352
This is a quarterly journal for health professionals featuring the
best of nutritional research and clinical trials.
One year subscription is $55 (U.S. funds)
and $58.85 (Canadian funds)
Two year subscription is $100 (U.S. funds)
and $107 (Canadian funds)

## Reference books

Here is a list of books available through
IMPAKT Communications (1-800-477-2995):

*Beating Cancer with Nutrition*
by Patrick Quillin, Ph.D., $16.95
(Price includes shipping and handling.)
Clinically proven and easy-to-follow strategies to dramatically
improve your quality and quantity of life and chances for a
complete remission. Dr. Quillin shows that the cancer patient
will thrive or wither, live or die, based upon being able to change
the conditions that allow cancer to thrive.
(Paperback, 254 pages)

*Cancer and Nutrition:*
*A Ten-Point Plan to Reduce Your Risk of Getting Cancer*
by Charles B. Simone, M.D., $14.95
(Price includes shipping and handling.)
With no exotic formulas and no expensive regimen, Dr. Simone provides the average person with a realistic program that can help save his or her life. Learn what foods to eat, what exercises to do, and what supplements to take.
(Paperback, 338 pages)

*Breast Cancer: What You Should Know (But May Not Be Told)*
*About Prevention, Diagnosis, and Treatment*
by Steve Austin, N.D., and Cathy Hitchcock, M.S.W. $18.95
(Price includes priority mail shipping.)
A husband-and-wife team, Hitchcock and Austin walk you step-by-step through each part of diagnosis, treatment (both conventional and alternative), and prevention (including prevention of a recurrence.) Interwoven with all this information, Cathy shares her personal story as a breast cancer survivor.
(Paperback, 336 pages)

*Preventing and Reversing Osteoporosis*
by Alan R. Gaby, M.D., $16.95
(Price includes shipping and handling.)
Dr. Gaby, one of the foremost authorities on nutritional and natural medicine, offers practical advice on osteoporosis that substantially increases a woman's chance for maintaining and even regaining normal bone mass.
(Paperback, 304 pages)

*Questions and Answers on Family Health*
by Jan de Vries, $10.95
(Price includes shipping and handling.)
No home should be without this valuable reference book.
In this book, European researcher Jan de Vries uses his vast wealth of experience to answer hundreds of questions which have consistently been asked of him over the years.
(Paperback, 280 pages)

*Healing Power of Herbs*
by Michael T. Murray, N.D., $17.95
(Price includes shipping and handling.)
Newly revised and updated, this handy reference book contains the latest scientific information on the world's most important medicinal plants. Here, in one of the most up-to-date and carefully researched books on botanical medicine, Dr. Michael Murray shares with you the latest scientific findings about the power and efficacy of medicinal herbs.
(Paperback, 410 pages)

*Natural Alternatives to Over-the-Counter and Prescription Drugs*
by Michael T. Murray, N.D., $30.00
(Price includes priority mail shipping.)
The first reference book to list natural alternatives to almost every common medicine. Including safe, natural alternatives to Tagamet, Prednisone, Zantac, and 207 other prescription drugs, as well as natural alternatives to over-the-counter drugs used to treat many common ailments.
(Hardcover, 383 pages)

*Encyclopedia of Natural Medicine*
by Michael T. Murray, N.D., $21.95
(Price includes priority mail shipping.)
Over 600 pages of the most comprehensive information on maintaining good health, preventing illness, and treating disease naturally and safely! Drawing on the best of centuries-old wisdom and modern knowledge and supported with the latest scientific investigation, the *Encyclopedia of Natural Medicine* is an important reference for anyone seeking to live a vibrant, healthful life.
(Paperback, 622 pages)

*Dr. Whitaker's Guide to Natural Healing*
by Julian Whitaker, M.D., $26.00
(Price includes priority mail shipping.)
Instead of focusing on disease, Dr. Whitaker's book is a blueprint for healthful living. He provides a comprehensive road map for wellness by covering:

- Prescriptions for optimal health that focus on prevention and wellness.
- Natural remedies and prevention techniques for nearly 100 specific health conditions, ranging from the common cold to hyperactivity and learning disorders.
- How you can create your own, truly effective healthcare system.
- And so much more!

(Hardcover, 417 pages)

*Flavor Without Fat*
by best selling author Jan McBarron, M.D. $17.95
(Price includes shipping and handling.)
Decrease your risk of cancer and heart disease while achieving your ideal weight. Eat healthy without sacrificing flavor by following the many practical, easy-to-use recipes included in this book.
(Paperback, 312 pages)

*Guess What Came To Dinner*
by Ann Louise Gittleman, M.D. $11.95
(Price includes shipping and handling.)
Are you having difficulty shaking off an illness? Are you suffering from chronic fatigue? Do you have a health problem your doctor can't identify? Parasites in your body may be the cause. Is there anything you can do to protect yourself and your family from this very real epidemic? Yes, there is. Top nutritionist Ann Louise Gittleman has written an easy-to-understand guide that gives you all the information you need to guard against these unwelcome organisms.
(Paperback, 194 pages)

*Alternative Medicine, The Definitive Guide*
by Deepak Chopra, M.D.. $55.00
(Price includes shipping and handling.)
It's a big book that can make a big difference in your family's health. *Alternative Medicine's* 1068 pages are filled with easy to understand information that is up-to-date.Whether the condition is cancer or a cold, you'll learn effective alternative ways to treat it, both by your-

self and with the help of healthcare professionals. To make this book as useful as possible, at the end of every chapter you'll find listings of how to find expert help with a specific condition or therapy, along with addresses and phone numbers. And you'll find a list of additional reading on the subject.
(Hardcover, 1068 pages)

You can order any of these books by calling 1-800-477-2995 or sending a check or money order to IMPAKT Communications, Inc., P.O. Box 12496, Green Bay, WI 54307-2496. *With every book order, you will receive a FREE Dr. Whitaker's Guide to Natural Healing (a $23 value) if you mention that you have a copy of the Help Yourself book!*

*Alternative Medicine: Expanding Medical Horizons*
a report to the National Institutes of Health on Alternative Medical Systems and Practices in the United States
$25 (Paperback, 372 pages)
Credit card purchases can call (202) 512-1800 or send a check or money order to Superintendent of Documents, P.O. Box 371954, Pittsburgh, PA 15250-7954

*Take Charge of Your Body* by Carolyn DeMarco, M.D.
$26.97 Canadian funds (expect a 40 percent savings when paying with a United States MasterCard or VISA)
To order call 1-800-387-4761

*Alternative Medicine Yellow Pages*
compiled by the Burton Goldberg Group
$12.95 (Paperback, 240 pages)
1-800-720-6363

*Healing Secrets from the Bible* by Patrick Quillin, Ph.D., C.N.S.
$14.95 (Paperback, 171 pages)
The Leader Co., Inc.
931 N. Main No. 101
N. Canton, OH 44720
(216) 494-6988 FAX (216) 494-6989

## Organizations

- Academy for Guided Imagery
  P.O. Box 2070
  Mill Valley, CA  94942
  1-800-726-2070
  FAX (415) 389-9342

- American Association of Acupuncture and Oriental Medicine
  433 Front Street
  Catasaugua, PA 18032
  (610) 266-1433 FAX (610) 264-2768
  For further information or a referral to a practitioner near you.

- American Association of Naturopathic Physicians
  2366 Eastlake Ave. East, Suite 322
  Seattle, WA 98102
  Referral Line (206) 323-7610
  To locate a naturopathic physician in the United States, send
  $5.00 for the AANP national referral directory.

- The American Osteopathic Association
  142 E. Ontario St.
  Chicago, IL 60611
  (800) 621-1773

- The American Board of Chelation Therapy
  1407-B North Wells
  Chicago, IL 60610
  (800) 356-2228 FAX (312) 266-3685
  For the names of board certified physicians practicing chelation therapy, send a self-addressed, stamped envelope.

- The American Botanical Council
  P.O. Box 201660
  Austin, TX 78720
  (512) 331-8868 FAX (512) 331-1924
  Provides information on herbs and herbal research.

- American College for Advancement in Medicine
  P.O. Box 3427
  Laguna Hills, CA 92654
  (800) 532-3688 outside CA (714) 583-7666 CA only

- National Center for Homeopathy
  801 North Fairfax, Suite 306
  Alexandria, VA 22314
  (703) 548-7790
  Provides a list of physicians who practice homeopathy.

- Institute of HeartMath
  P.O. Box 1463
  Boulder Creek, CA  95006
  (408) 338-8700 FAX (408) 338-9861

- International Academy of Nutrition and Preventive Medicine
  P.O. Box 18433
  Asheville, NC 28814
  (704) 258-3243
  Provides a list of health professionals who use nutrition and
  preventive medicine.

- Wellness Referral Network Inc.
  (800) 520-WELL
  Provides free information and referral to providers who focuses
  on nutrition, prevention and complementary medicine.

## Natural medicine political information

Citizen's For Health
P.O. Box 368
Tacoma, WA 98401
(206) 922-2457
This is a nonprofit natural medicine advocacy group.

## Natural medicine insurance

American Medical Security
P.O. Box 10974-0974
Green Bay, WI 54307-9868
1-800-232-5432
Ask about the HealthCareChoice$ holistic health insurance plan.

## Nutritional supplement manufacturers

Enzymatic Therapy
1-800-783-2286
For a free *Essential Formulas for Health* guide and a list of health
food stores in your area, call between 8 a.m. and 5 p.m. (CST)
Monday through Friday.

Carlson Labs
1-800-323-4141
For information about a store in your area that carries Carlson Labs
products.

Flora
1-800-498-3610
For information about a store in your area that carries Flora
products.

Alta Health
California (818) 796-1047
Outside California 1-800-423-4155

## On death and dying

National Hospice Organization
1901 North Moore St., Suite 901
Arlington, VA  22209
(703) 243-5900
Hospice Helpline:  1-800-658-8898

# GLOSSARY

## Natural Medicine Terminology

### Acupuncture

This procedure uses needles to penetrate and stimulate specific points throughout the body. The purpose of acupuncture is to restore normal body function and renew the body's energetic balance.

### Ayurvedic medicine

Originating in India, ayurvedic medicine is an ancient form of treatment that involves diet, detoxification, exercise, herbal medicine and meditation. Ayurvedic medicine is effective for the treatment of a wide variety of chronic health conditions.

### Biofeedback

This type of training teaches the patient how to consciously control their autonomic (involuntary) nervous system by using biofeedback devices which sound a tone when changes in pulse, blood pressure, brain waves, and muscle contractions occur. Biofeedback training is most commonly used to alleviate stress, migraine headaches, asthma, and high blood pressure.

### Chelation therapy

Chelation therapy is a medical process that uses an intravenous solution to remove heavy metals and toxins from the blood. It is commonly used to reverse atherosclerosis and as an alternative to bypass surgery and angioplasty. Chelation therapy has also been shown to reduce high blood pressure and help reverse age-related degenerative diseases.

### Detoxification

This type of therapy helps to rid the body of chemicals and pollutants and can also facilitate a return to health. Forms of detoxification therapy include fasting, massage, hydrotherapy, and juicing.

### Guided imagery

This type of meditation capitalizes on the power of the mind by creating mental pictures that help stimulate a positive physical response. It is commonly used to help stimulate the immune system, reduce stress, and slow heart rate.

### Herbal medicine
Having an extensive history of usage throughout the world, herbal medicine uses plant substances as medicine. Research has shown herbal medicines to be effective in a wide range of conditions.

### Homeopathy
Homeopathic medicine uses minute traces of a medicinal substance to stimulate the healing processes of the body in order to restore health and normal body function. Homeopathy is used extensively in England, Europe, Mexico, and India.

### Hypnotherapy
This is a method used to tap into a person's unconscious mind to help facilitate the treatment of a variety of conditions including depression, stress, anxiety, obesity, and eating disorders.

### Naturopathy
This is a system of medicine based upon natural principles of health and a respect for the healing power of nature. Naturopathy, also known as naturopathic medicine, utilizes therapies such as diet, herbal medicine, hydrotherapy, lifestyle counselling, acupuncture, and homeopathy to help the body heal itself.

### Osteopathy
Osteopathic physicians use body manipulation, physical, medicinal, and surgical techniques to restore good health and balance within their patients. This is known as osteopathy, which is designed to remove any internal or external abnormalities. It is recognized as a standard method or system of medical and surgical care.

### Holistic
According to Webster's dictionary, holistic means "relating to or concerned with wholes or with complete systems rather than with the analysis of, treatment of, or dissection into parts." Holistic medicine attempts to treat both the mind and the body. Holistic healthcare is a system of treatment that takes into consideration all aspects of health. Holistic theory suggests that we are much more than the sum of our individual parts. Treating illness holistically means exploring all

aspects of the human condition, attempting to analyze the true cause of illness rather than treat only the symptoms.

### Natural medicine

Treatments that are effective, natural, nontoxic and least invasive fall under the category of natural medicine. These treatments can involve diet and lifestyle changes, botanical and nutritional supplements, homeopathic medicines, acupuncture, and many others. People who use natural medicine treatments believe that the human body, when given the opportunity, has the ability to heal itself when it is provided the proper tools. Natural medicine treats the whole person and trusts in the healing power of nature.

### Therapeutic nutrition

Using the diet as therapy is a key treatment method of many natural medicine practitioners. "There is an ever increasing body of knowledge that supports the use of whole foods and nutritional supplements in the maintenance of health and treatment of disease," according to natural medicine researcher Dr. Michael Murray. Therapeutic nutrition provides specific nutrients the body needs to help defend itself from dangerous illness. It is believed that most common conditions can be treated effectively with dietary measures alone including arthritis, asthma, hypertension, PMS, etc. It has also been shown that nearly 80 percent to 90 percent of all cancers are produced as a result of dietary and nutritional practices, lifestyle (smoking, alcohol, etc.), chemicals and other environmental factors. Therapeutic nutrition attempts to address the areas that are nutritionally deficient or lacking and fills in the gaps via diet and dietary supplements.

### Dietary supplements

A product containing one or more nutrient (i.e. vitamin, mineral, amino acid, etc.) is a dietary supplement. Dietary supplements are also called nutritional supplements and are used to help complement the diet as a means of prevention or treatment of illness. Dietary supplements are one method of treatment used by many holistic healthcare providers.

### Vitamins

Vitamins are organic substances essential in the regulation of many metabolic processes in the human body. Vitamins are found in foods and sometimes produced within the body. Vitamin supplements are designed to provide the body with a specific vitamin that may be deficient in the diet or may be needed in higher dosages due to health status.

### Standardized botanical extracts

A botanical extract is an herb that is used for medicinal purposes. It is estimated that about 25 percent of all prescription drugs in the United States contain active constituents obtained from plants. Botanical extracts have a long history of use as herbal medicines. Standardization is a scientific technique used to ensure quality and consistency among botanical products. Botanical extracts standardized for a specific active constituent ensure each and every capsule has the same potency to provide the user with consistent results.

### Amino acids

Amino acids are considered the building blocks of protein. There are 22 separate amino acids: 13 can be manufactured in the body and the other 9 are available through dietary protein. Nutritional supplements often contain certain amino acids. Specific amino acids work closely with specific body functions. For example, L-tryptophan is an essential amino acid that influences brain function. Amino acids are available within dietary supplement formulations or as separate products.

### Glandular extract therapy

Glandular therapy uses extracts as an important form of medicine. Glandular therapy believes that like heals like. For example, if your liver needs therapeutic support, you may benefit from eating beef liver. Modern glandular therapy, however, uses concentrated glandular extracts, which contain active hormones and enzymes. Glands commonly used in extracts include the pituitary, thyroid, thymus, pancreas, and adrenal. Other organs, such as heart, spleen, liver, etc., can also be used as glandular extracts. Glandular extracts can be sold separately or as part of a dietary supplement formulation.

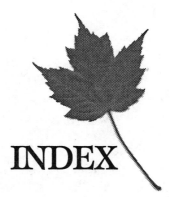

# INDEX

# IMPAKT
**Communications**
**P.O. Box 12496**
**Green Bay, WI  54307-2496**
**1-800-477-2995**

Subscribe to *Health Counselor* magazine for one year and receive a **FREE** *Dr. Whitaker's Guide to Natural Healing*—that's a $23 value! This hard-cover book by nationally recognized wellness doctor, Julian Whitaker, M.D., features advice on natural remedies for nearly 100 specific health conditions.

*Health Counselor* magazine provides accurate, up-to-date information on vitamins, minerals, herbs, and other nutrients. Each issue features scientific information on natural therapies for a wide variety of conditions. This is a full-color, bi-monthly magazine that only costs $18 per year (six issues). Subscribe today and receive your **FREE** book!

**Method of payment**

❏ Check   ❏ MasterCard   ❏ VISA   ❏ American Express

Name:_____

Address:_____

City, State,Zip: _____

Phone:_____

Name on card:_____

Signature:_____

Card Number:_____

Exp. Date:_____